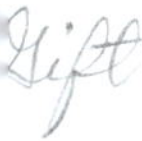

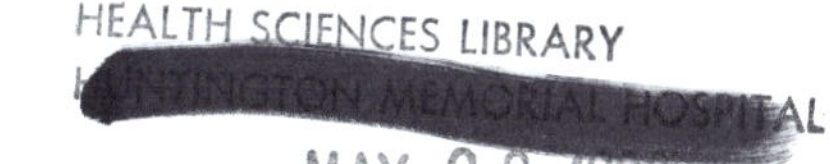

The Business of Nursing

AONE Leadership Series

American Organization
of Nurse Executives

AHA books are published by American Hospital Publishing, Inc.,
an American Hospital Association company

A • O N E

This publication is designed to provide accurate and authoritative information in regard to the subject matter covered. It is sold with the understanding that neither the author nor the publisher is engaged in rendering legal, accounting, or other professional service. If legal advice or other expert assistance is required, the services of a competent professional person should be sought.

The views expressed in this publication are strictly those of the author and do not necessarily represent official positions of the American Hospital Association.

Library of Congress Cataloging-in-Publication Data

The business of nursing / American Organization of Nurse Executives.
    p.   cm.—(AONE leadership series)
  Includes bibliographical references.
  ISBN 1-55648-151-9
  1. Nursing services—Administration. I. American Organization of Nurse Executives. II. Series.
  [DNLM: 1. Nursing. 2. Nurse Administrators. 3. Nursing Services——organization & administration. WY 16 B979 1995]
RT89.B87 1995
362.1'73'068—dc20
DNLM/DLC
for Library of Congress   95-47785
                                         CIP

Catalog no. 154153

©1996 by American Hospital Publishing, Inc.,
an American Hospital Association company

Printed in the USA

AHA is a service mark of the American Hospital Association used under license by American Hospital Publishing, Inc.

Text set in Sabon

3M—2/96—0433

Audrey Kaufman, Senior Editor
Lee Benaka, Editor
Peggy DuMais, Production Coordinator
Marcia Bottoms, Executive Editor

Contents

List of Figures and Tables

About the Authors

Marjorie Beyers, PhD, RN, FAAN, is executive director of the American Organization of Nurse Executives, Chicago. Previously, Dr. Beyers was vice-president, nursing and allied health systems, at Mercy Health Services, Farmington Hills, Michigan, where she provided leadership for systemwide nursing and allied health services. She has published extensively and consulted in the areas of nursing administration and quality issues in health care. In addition, Dr. Beyers has presented more than 200 lectures to hospitals, nursing schools, and professional organizations nationwide. She was the first recipient of the Roy Woodham Visiting Fellowship Award for research in the areas of financing, organization, and delivery of health services in multi-institutional systems.

Richard Brock, MA, CNAA, RN, is a manager, health care consulting practice, southwest region for Ernst and Young, LLP. Mr. Brock has been an active member of the American Organization of Nurse Executives for 15 years, serving as a consultant and director for membership services. Prior to his consulting work, Mr. Brock was a nurse executive at Santa Barbara Cottage Hospital (California) and Los Angeles County/USC Medical Center.

Geraldene Felton, EdD, BSN, MSN, RN, FAAN, is professor and dean of the College of Nursing at the University of Iowa, Iowa City. A retired Army Nurse Corps officer, Dr. Felton was deputy director of the Walter Reed Institute of Research department of nursing (Washington, DC) and has held faculty positions at the University of Hawaii and Georgetown University. Prior to her work at the University of Iowa, she was professor and dean of nursing at the Oakland University School of Nursing in Rochester, Michigan. Dr. Felton has held many positions in associations and organizations, including chair of the National Institutes of Health Nursing Research Study Section and president of the American Association of Colleges of Nursing. In addition, she has conducted numerous research and training projects;

written many book chapters, monographs, and articles; and given over 100 presentations.

Katherine R. Jones, PhD, RN, FAAN, is associate professor, division of nursing systems, at the University of Michigan's School of Nursing, Ann Arbor. Dr. Jones also serves as adjunct nursing administrator at the University of Michigan Medical Center, where she conducts clinical and organizational outcomes research. Previously, she was a faculty member at the University of California, Los Angeles, School of Nursing, and in the University of Florida's (Gainesville) health and hospital administration program. In addition, Dr. Jones completed a postdoctoral fellowship in health finance at Johns Hopkins University, Baltimore.

Julianne M. Morath, MS, RN, is system vice-president, quality, for Allina Health System, Minnetonka, Minnesota. She previously served as vice-president of patient care at Abbott Northwestern Hospital, Minneapolis. Ms. Morath is a frequent speaker on the subjects of systems thinking, community health, labor management, and human dynamics.

Joan M. Rimar, MSN, RN, is special projects coordinator, division of nursing, at Yale–New Haven Hospital, New Haven, Connecticut. She was formerly a pediatric nurse manager at Yale–New Haven Hospital.

Diana J. Weaver, DNS, RN, FAAN, is senior vice-president, patient services, at Yale–New Haven Hospital, New Haven, Connecticut. She previously was associate hospital director, director of nursing, University of Kentucky Hospital, Lexington. Ms. Weaver served as president of American Organization of Nurse Executives from 1995 to 1996.

Preface

The Business of Nursing initially was intended to be a resource of best practices for executive nurses to use in creating integrated health care delivery systems. Its content and case studies were to help nurses bring about change in their own settings. However, as the project took on a life of its own, its intent shifted. It began to focus on the change processes and innovations needed to adjust to a new health care culture in which considerable variation exists in each care delivery model's organization, structure, process, and policies. Therefore, rather than provide models, this book shares insights on how to bring about changes in philosophy, attitude, and approach. Its authors discuss how the new health care delivery environment requires shifts in thinking about nursing care; new competencies for education and executive practice; and new relationships with colleagues both within and outside the nursing department.

The Business of Nursing is about the vision of the future, the business of integrated health care delivery systems, and the process of change. Because the approaches to making the transition to this future are not yet mature enough to force into categorizations useful for benchmarking, it would be a disservice to include them at this stage. Rather, this book offers a preliminary discussion of what lies ahead.

People we talked to about this project expressed great interest in what was meant by the "business" of nursing care. Was the term *business* being used to mean getting work accomplished or to mean reducing cost and realizing profit? Everyone agreed that the nurse executive role is changing in not only resources available for care delivery but also performance expectations and relationships. Although most people accepted the notion that nursing care has to change in synchrony with health care, many had difficulty accepting that its practice should be treated as a business. They found this notion contrary to time-honored beliefs that human services should be immune from economic concerns. For many, such beliefs override the growing acceptance that health care systems are being "corporatized." In corporate thinking, any service of value has a price. Although certainly nurse executives agree that nursing care is a valued human service, there is lively debate about whether it should have a price. Thus, the a priori issue is: How does the practice of nursing fit into the business of health care? Tensions currently are building to clarify nursing, both as a service and as a business.

The Role of Nursing in Integrated Health Care Delivery Systems

There is no question that nursing services have been, and will continue to be, integral to health care delivery. Nurses have the capability to serve clients in a vast array of health services such as health promotion, acute care, long-term and chronic care, hospice care, and community interventions. Nursing also has considerable flexibility and a record of adaptation to change. In all the previously mentioned settings, nursing has adapted to changing resource availability, new demands triggered by social and economic changes, and new environments and cultures. Nurse executives have become master resource managers, with the ability to respond to stringent demands for efficiency and efficacy. However, nursing's capability to create new services and to innovate has been underutilized. And these are competencies that are relevant to any type of business.

The debate, then, is not about whether nursing services are necessary or add value. Rather, it is steeped in philosophical groundings: whether nursing should be treated as a business entity or an essential human service. In either case, nursing care must be recognized and appreciated for its worth, value, and price in every setting where health care is delivered, including the integrated health care delivery systems.

Moving from delivering care in a specific type of setting such as a hospital or the home to an integrated health care delivery system with "seamless" care is challenging. Attitudes, values, regulations, and past practices can be either barriers to or facilitators of change. Nurse executives need to understand why these changes must be accomplished, and must be able to articulate them and the vision they represent. They must become involved in determining not only the future direction of health care but also how it is to be accomplished.

Integration is the creation of the new. In many cases, the new is created only by dispelling boundaries and barriers between and among entities such as hospital, home, and ambulatory and community-based health services. Nurses are proving their worth because they are among the more mobile of health professionals, equally effective in every care delivery setting. When they perceive that their services are essential to health care delivery in every setting, they will have the confidence to lead the innovations toward integration.

Moving toward integration also means moving resources and supplies, people, and processes. Appropriate resources and supplies for care are essential to quality functioning in any setting. *Integration* means moving the care to the customer, a move that requires inevitable changes in both the organization and processes of care delivery. The new organization and processes must support the clinical care, which is increasingly visible as integrated health care delivery systems are developed.

Although the vision of integrated health care delivery systems is clear, the worldview of nursing services within those systems is less so. However, some trends are evident. For example, nurses in executive practice are becoming involved in designing health care delivery services and systems. They are working with health care teams to implement care delivery. The context and concepts in which this work is grounded are continuity of care in the lifetime continuum and managed care financing. This work is taking place in new organizational forms in which individuality and uniqueness are more characteristic than not. However, there is no emerging template for organizing the structure and defining the processes for integrated health care systems and delivery. What is emerging is that the redesign efforts are predicated on concepts and principles of change, processes such as total quality management and continuous improvement, and innovative new consolidations and alliances, including new relationships between communities and health care providers.

The Business of Nursing provides information that, if integrated into nurse executive behaviors, should enhance the practice of nursing care. The values of nursing can be enhanced in the new health care system if nurses in executive practice are capable of sorting out the essence of nursing from the change processes that influence the practice of nursing. Thus, this book offers the following perspective:

> The core of nursing service is threaded throughout the health care delivery system. Organizational and system factors that comprise the environment for practice should be viewed as supporting customer service.

Every nurse must understand and value nursing care to effectively move in concert with the evolution of integrated health care delivery systems. Whatever the perspective, the business of nursing remains patient care.

Marjorie Beyers, PhD, RN, FAAN
Executive Director
American Organization of Nurse Executives

December 1995

Acknowledgments

Nurses in executive practice are moving forward to define new ways to deliver patient care in integrated health care delivery systems. This book is a reflection of the force of change and the impact of change on health care organizations and the people who work in them. The notion of a book about the business of nursing care was brought to life by Audrey Kaufman and through the participation of members of the American Organization of Nurse Executives (AONE), who provided ideas and concepts, reviewed manuscripts, and kept the content grounded in reality. The assistance and insights of Rhonda Anderson, Pam Bromley, and Diana Weaver were especially helpful. *The Business of Nursing* is both a recognition of the expertise of AONE members and a statement of commitment to excellence in practice.

Introduction

The Business of Nursing reflects the complexity of changes in health care, the impact of change on patients and families, and the new challenges facing nurses in executive practice as they respond to change and develop new systems of care delivery. The content of this book was selected to provide an overview of future trends, insights about the change process, strategies for decision making in complex environments, real-life change experiences (through a case study), and perspectives on the future practice and education of nurses in executive roles. Each chapter in this book provides information and thoughtful prodding about nursing issues and challenges.

Chapter 1 discusses future trends and directions in nurse executive practice by presenting basic assumptions about the future. The first assumption is that health care is moving from a needs-driven to a resource-driven mindset. Resources must equate positively with significant patient outcomes. The second assumption is that the work of patient care is being positioned differently in integrated health care delivery systems. The resulting gestalt allows nurses in executive practice to actualize new imperatives for meeting patient care needs throughout the continuum of care. The third assumption is that both the clinical practice and education of caregivers is directly influenced by technology and the timeliness of information.

Chapters 2 and 3 offer two approaches to change that are both necessary to meet current challenges. Chapter 2 focuses on relationships and the importance of dealing with responses to change and building the grounding for new realities. The importance of working with staff nurses to facilitate the shift from traditional paradigms to new paradigms is presented. The main point of the chapter is that nurses now offer value to health care delivery because of their critical-thinking capabilities. Chapter 3 presents the perspective of data-driven decision making. Seemingly in contrast to the relationships approach of chapter 2, chapter 3 discusses how to ask and answer a cogent question: What is the cost–benefit of providing care in patients' homes rather than hospitals or nursing homes? Chapter 3 argues that a data-driven approach yields considerable information that in early stages of change may add complexity to the issues while also providing insight into the problems. The chapter also contends that a great deal of change currently occurring in health care is based on projections and visions rather than on data that prove cost–benefit effectiveness. Both chapters imply that organizational learning is a key to future success.

Chapter 4 illustrates how vision and responses to change are brought together through innovations. The chapter's account of pacesetting innovation at Abbott Northwestern Hospital, Minneapolis, shows how one health care system adapted to a market-driven environment with nurses as independent partners. Chapter 4 provides insights into emerging issues such as whether nursing or patient care can truly be standardized. The chapter acknowledges that the reductionistic and mechanistic application of business practices to health care can be limiting, and contends that high-quality customer service in health care demands customization or, in nursing terms, individualized patient care. This chapter's message is that quality is the key goal, and its achievement requires technical excellence, the capacity for diagnostic and therapeutic care, and positive personal experiences with care.

The final two chapters in this book look at future challenges in nurse executive practice. Based on the assumption that nurse executive practice is embedded in the context of changing health care delivery, the science of nursing administration practice is being transformed. Chapter 5 reflects on selected patterns of change that have occurred thus far and some of the key views of nursing practice and care delivery. Recommendations for how to frame future challenges and imperatives are also provided. Chapter 6 describes what must be accomplished to prepare nursing leaders for the future. Changes in health care financing have implications for the roles, responsibilities, and practices in all health care disciplines such as nursing. Insights are influenced by the vision of shaping integrated health care delivery systems that improve access to care and the capability to promote health as well as provide care along the lifetime continuum.

Because many new terms are used in today's health care dialogues, some of the more frequently used new terms, as well as time-honored terms with new interpretations, are collected in the glossary at the end of this book. These terms provide further insights into the complexities of integrated health care delivery systems and managed care.

Chapter 1

Understanding the Patient Care Executive's Changing Role and Responsibilities

Diana J. Weaver, DNS, RN, FAAN,
and Joan M. Rimar, MSN, RN

In Victor Hugo's novel *Les Misérables,* the former thief Jean Valjean is confronted with a moral and ethical dilemma. After having been saved by a priest from inevitable arrest and imprisonment and having built a successful life for himself as mayor of a small town, he discovers that his relentless pursuer, Chief Inspector Javêrt, has mistakenly arrested another man for his crime. Valjean's dilemma is clear: He can remain silent and continue to do good work among the villagers who have come to depend on him, or he can come forward to save the innocent man at the cost of depriving the villagers of his leadership. Valjean's dilemma is familiar—whether to act for the good of one or for the good of many. Like Valjean, health care professionals wrestle with this dilemma and frequently understand that serving both goals is rarely possible.

The decision of whether to meet the health care needs of the many versus the one is difficult for clinicians who are comfortable practicing within a needs-driven, rather than a resource-sensitive, framework. And although present-day patient care executives understand the need to embrace the scarce-resource model and its implications for planning and allocating patient care, they also recognize that moving from the mode of *do all you can for all patients* to that of *thoughtfully and critically allocate resources* demands a new way of thinking that may conflict with long-held values.

This chapter presents a brief historical perspective of health care delivery in the United States, and describes the current status of patient care costs. It then discusses the patient care executive's role in helping clinicians work within the resource-sensitive framework.[1]

Historical Perspective of Care Delivery in the United States

Since first opening in the U.S., hospitals have aimed to provide all appropriate care for patients with little regard to either resource consumption or ability to pay. As biotechnological advances and clinical knowledge have expanded, patients have been treated with ever-multiplying goods and services. In the past, patient care took place in large wards where one nurse attended to the simple hygiene, nutrition, and mobility needs of as many as 15 to 20 patients; today, each critically ill patient is cared for around the clock by one and sometimes two registered nurses (RNs) in a private or semiprivate setting.

In the past, little attention was paid to the financial impact of resource consumption or the relationship between resource use and patient outcome or societal impact. Staff nurse concern with the cost of supplies was minimal, and the contribution of the use of available items to patient progress or outcomes was rarely examined critically. Nor did hospital administrators consistently compare patient outcomes on similar units with significantly different expenditures.

Over the years, technological advances and consumer willingness to pay have caused the simple tools of yesterday, such as the stethoscope, the thermometer, and the blood pressure cuff, to be replaced by the complex, highly specialized, and often computerized machines found in hospitals today. However, paradoxically, whereas the introduction of new technology into other businesses reduces the cost of labor, its introduction into health care often increases the cost of patient care. People, frequently RNs, are needed to watch monitors, read gauges, record data, and care for the devices to keep them ticking, timing, and ever engaged.

The rising cost of health care and the impact of that cost on the gross domestic product (GDP) has caused Americans to begin to demand that health care institutions account for the cost of the care they provide. Said differently, resources used must equate positively and significantly to patient outcomes.

Current Cost of Patient Care

Today, health care costs represent approximately 15 percent of the GDP. Economists estimate that if their growth goes unchecked, health care costs will represent almost 16 percent of the GDP by the turn of the century.[2] This would be an unsustainable burden on the U.S. economy.

Many Americans relate the total cost of health care to the dollars spent on hospital care, because hospital care spotlights costs associated with drugs, equipment, physician services, overhead, and daily labor. Although this perception is understandable, it is narrow and incorrect. What is not evident to the public are all the other costs that must be factored into the total cost of care delivery, including associated medical education, pharmaceutical and technological research and development, escalating regulatory mandates, marketing efforts, and the impact of lifestyle and environmental factors on health status.

In the past five to ten years, because of concerns about rising costs, the private-payment sector has shifted its mentality from that of paying for all charges to that of providing fixed dollars for different episodes of treatment. In part, this shift mirrors government's approach to controlling health care costs for the Medicare population that occurred with the introduction of the diagnosis-related group (DRG) system. Another impetus for the change was the business sector's realization that employee health care costs were claiming an ever-increasing percentage of its profits.

Until recently, health care institutions were able to compensate for the lower Medicare reimbursement rate by shifting the cost of the unfinanced care to those patients covered by private-payer sources. This widely acknowledged and accepted pea-and-shell game fundamentally insulated all stakeholders, including patients and health care providers, from the real cost associated with the health care system. However, revenues began to decrease as private payers cut reimbursement rates significantly and as hospitals negotiated further discounts to attract patients. Therefore, cost shifting is no longer possible because hospitals do not have dollars to redirect to cover uninsured or underinsured patients.

Business concepts such as scarce-resource allocation, cost–benefit analysis, and opportunity cost can provide a logical framework in which to address issues associated with the cost of patient care. The concept of scarce-resource allocation compels one to ask, "What is the best use of our resources given limited resource availability, patients' needs and desires, and potential outcomes?" Cost–benefit analysis prompts questions such as, "Do the total benefits (outputs) to the patient, health care organization, or society exceed the total costs (inputs) of the proposed program, procedure, or initiative?" The concept of opportunity cost is elaborated by Russell in the following manner: "The opportunity cost of devoting resources to a particular use is defined as the loss of the benefits the resources could have produced had they been put to their best use—the lost opportunity to invest in that alternative."[3]

However, the business production model of input, throughput, and output (see figure 1-1) can result in a simplistic and incomplete framework for managing clinical resources because of the profusion of factors that affect health and, consequently, health care. The model of a resource information

Figure 1-1.   Business Production Model

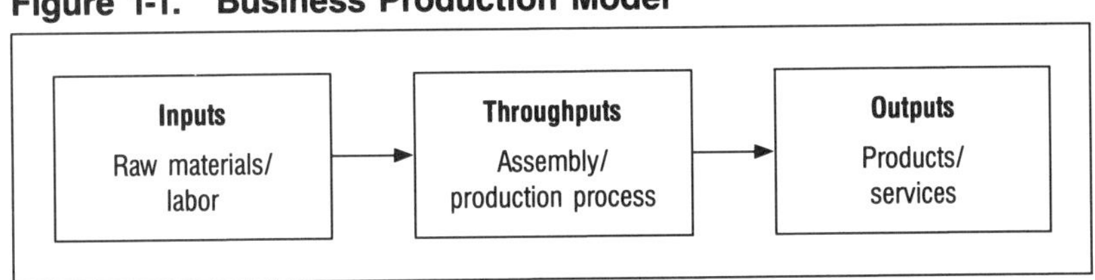

management system shown in figure 1-2 creates a more appropriate framework because it demonstrates the complexity of the clinical, operational, and financial inputs, throughputs, and outputs associated with hospital care.

Many factors affect health care costs, including caregiver education and training; availability and use of technology; and timeliness of interventions. Patient variables in the equation include comorbidities and their effect on response to therapy.

Caregiver Education and Training

The education of caregivers also augurs against managing patient care institutions in a businesslike manner. As stated previously, nurses, physicians, and others have been educated to value the individual and have progressed in their professions with the notion that whatever a patient needs must be made available. To accept any less has been counter to the American ethos that values individualism and heroism. The curricula of health care professionals contain little business or ethics education, and our schools have been slow to instruct students in the solid ethical principles that underlie good business practices.

Moreover, *paternalism* (making people do what is good for them or, conversely, preventing people from doing what is bad for them), particularly in the education of physicians, has created a power differential between system and patient.[4] This power differential is realized when the system does not make complete information on the cost and potential value of planned interventions and resource use available to the patient. Health care professionals must more consistently seek to establish the value that people attach to preventing illness or curing or ameliorating the effects of disease by negotiating the health care services to be rendered given the limited available resources. We must ask what people are willing to pay in terms of both dollars and intangibles such as lifestyle changes and emotional commitment in order to obtain desired outcomes. In fairness to physicians and other caregivers, the research base to support a new model of care delivery that functions within a scarce-resource framework has been lacking and presents a challenge to those seeking to manage health care as a business. This is true for several reasons but predominantly because the complexity and multifactorial nature of care does not lend itself to simple analysis or a linear approach to decision making.

Technology and Timeliness

The questions of which intervention to use and when to use it can significantly affect the cost of health care. For example, the left ventricular assist device (LVAD), a relatively new technology, can prolong life for the seriously ill individual who is awaiting heart transplantation. Application of

Figure 1-2. Resource Information Management System Model

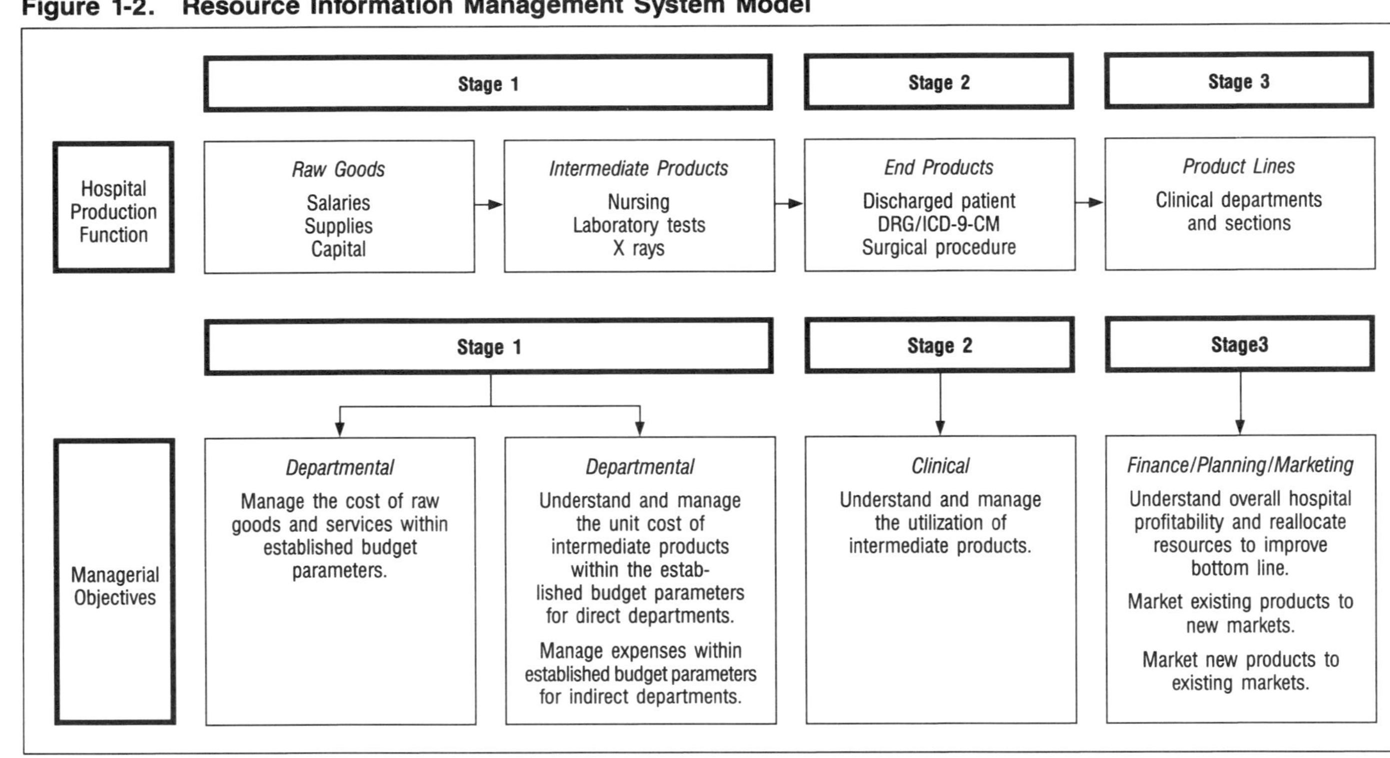

Source: Adapted by Stephen Allegretto, Yale–New Haven Hospital, New Haven, Connecticut, from *Transition I—A Functional Overview,* a 1989 manual developed by Transition Systems, Inc., Boston.

this technology is costly, but its potential to improve patients' outcomes has increased demand for the LVAD. The timeliness of LVAD placement affects the cost of care because too-early or too-late placement results in avoidable, noncontributory costs through inefficient use of resources.

The Effective Patient Care Executive Role and Responsibilities

Balancing the cost of care and the availability and consumption of myriad treatment and service options complicates nursing's mission to provide high-quality care to all patients. But with the emerging economic reality that health care resources must be treated as scarce commodities and that, frequently, the health care industry can do more for patients than it can afford to do, the patient care executive's responsibility to provide leadership and management of the core business of health care is remarkably clear. The successful patient care executive will use the fewest resources to ensure that his or her clients remain healthy, well-informed, and productive members of society for as long as possible. Ensuring access to efficient and effective patient care requires embracing a new paradigm and includes the following mandates:

- *Acquiring new tools and skills:* Systems thinking, business planning, acumen for new product development.
- *Assuming new functions:* Managing care across the entire continuum from wellness centers to home care and skilled nursing facilities.
- *Seeking, exploring, and seizing new opportunities:* Perhaps the most important mandate, this includes internalizing the knowledge that health care services will be delivered to patients across the lifespan and creating the appropriate environments and resources to provide desired services.

It also means that patient care executives must guide and support others, particularly clinicians, as they absorb the realities and implications of needing to consider opportunity costs.

To equip staff to manage the situation generated by emerging tension between traditional patient care values and the scarce-resource perspective, the successful patient care executive:

- Uses appropriate cost-accounting and decision support tools
- Educates staff and managers
- Supports clinical inquiry
- Moves toward best practices and standardizes practices whenever possible
- Uses continued improvement and continuous learning as a framework for improving care
- Shapes public and social health care policies

The following subsections discuss the patient care executive's responsibility with regard to supporting staff and manager education, clinical inquiry and creative problem solving, and use of research methodologies. The subsections also elaborate on the other elements of the preceding list.

The Responsibility to Educate

Patient care executives must ensure that both staff and managers understand the basic elements of budget development and budget management. In the past, nurse managers were provided little information on budget development yet were responsible for managing huge sums of money associated with labor and nonsalary resources such as equipment and supplies. Staff and managers understood little about the relationship between cost of care and clinical management of patients, including management directed by the strict and labor-intensive clinical standards they had developed themselves. Without a basic knowledge of budget development, it is impossible for caregivers to understand how to implement the least costly initiative chosen from an array of equal-quality patient management options.

It is up to the patient care executive to ensure that managers and staff have the tools needed to make decisions that support the delivery of cost-effective, high-quality care. The combination of today's financial information systems and the expertise of clinicians can produce the budgetary models needed to fill staff and managers' information void and provide a basis for sound decision making. Clinical standards that are supported by scientific evidence (when possible) and endorsed by clinical experts are valuable adjuncts to well-presented budget information in terms of producing desired outcomes. Consistent use of clinical standards and careful monitoring of associated outcomes provide an opportunity for identification and widespread institution of "best practices."

In addition, health care consumers need to understand the relationship between care, cost, and outcome. Current payment mechanisms promote indifference to these critical considerations by insulating consumers from the financial realities of care decisions and interventions. Possibly the greatest challenge to patient care executives in this particular area is to trust that everyone who directly or indirectly makes decisions that affect resource utilization understands the cost associated with redundant or nonvalued activities and acts with this knowledge in mind. A thoughtful analysis of all care-related activities and quality control initiatives is essential to address the cost–benefit issue, and such an initiative is best done by individual care providers, not patient care executives.

Finally, the patient care executive's education-related responsibilities reach far beyond the walls of his or her organization. The patient care executive must ensure the viability of his or her institution by anticipating and planning for change. Equally important, the patient care executive must appropriately and effectively advocate for patients and society in general. To accomplish these requirements, the executive must learn about current trends and act as an advocate and educator through the development of local, regional, and national health care policy.

The Responsibility to Support Clinical Inquiry and Creative Problem Solving

Perhaps one of the greatest contributions that the patient care executive can provide in the work setting is to support clinical inquiry at the provider level, in part to demonstrate the cost and benefit of service. Clinical inquiry begins with challenging care providers to question the value and meaning of current clinical practice within the care paradigm. Suggesting that staff ask why and why not in critically examining their practice is a good way to get the process started. Being able to ask these two questions is tantamount to challenging the status quo—a risky business. Often, giving tacit approval is the necessary first step in the process. For example, following are two studies that are looking at existing practices involving the possible overutilization (why) and underutilization (why not) of skillful nurses.

The first study came about as a result of a detected variability in the use of monitor watchers on units housing cardiac patients. Four patient care units with telemetry capability were using professional nurses as monitor watchers in a variety of patterns. The first unit used nurses as monitor watchers 24 hours a day, seven days a week; the second used them 16 hours a day; the third, 8 hours a day; and the fourth, not at all. Curiously, although the practice differences were known throughout the institution, no one had considered the impact of these practice differences on patient outcomes. Because the differences seemed to indicate the overutilization of skilled nurses, the initial inclination was to withdraw the monitor-watching service on all units. However, the nurse manager on the unit with the 24-hour availability was very concerned that withdrawal of this clinical support would have a negative effect on the patients there. She worked with a clinical nurse specialist and a faculty member from a nearby nursing school to develop a research proposal to study the effects of monitor watching on her patient population, and together they developed a controlled research proposal with funding awarded by an external source. The research is ongoing, and the results may provide needed information on the necessity of a resource-intensive approach to the clinical management of cardiac patients.

The second study seeks to quantify the intuitive knowledge of the triage nurse in predicting the need for hospital admission of patients seen in the emergency department (ED). It compares the physician's decision to admit a given patient with the triage nurse's prediction of that patient's admission. The triage nurse completes a prediction sheet on each patient and indicates whether he or she expects the patient to be admitted or discharged at the end of the ED visit. The confidence with which the nurse makes the prediction is marked on a Likert scale ranging from "not very confident" to "very confident." This type of study may allow for earlier identification of patients who need to be admitted and may demonstrate that the triage nurse currently is underutilized. If the correlation is positive and significant, the admission process can be initiated much sooner, and patients will receive appropriate interventions and be moved out of the busy and congested ED more quickly.

Another way to support clinical inquiry is to provide clinicians with data on resource cost and consumption and to identify patient outliers within a patient group. This often motivates clinicians to question why a segment of the population is different. To use data in this fashion requires that a solid cost-accounting system be in place and that the use of all resources be identified, tracked, and made available to the clinicians closest to the point of service, that is, the patient bedside.

Other supportive measures include ensuring that staff are given resources at the unit level to be able to "scratch a clinical itch." Such resources include relevant journals, in hard copy or on-line; available unit-based clinical experts or advanced practice nurses; and a regularly scheduled forum at the unit level where discussion of practice issues is a consistent agenda item. The catalyst for clinical inquiry might be practice variability across settings without grossly obvious differences in patient outcomes. Similarly, practice differences among primary nurses caring for the same patient population also provides impetus for why and why not questions.

The Responsibility to Support Use of Research Methodologies

To analyze clinical issues in a manner that adds to the knowledge base, staff require support in efforts to use accepted research methodologies. If an institution is unable to maintain a complete research department with full-time staff, clinical staff nevertheless can conduct research under the guidance of only one part-time researcher or with the cooperation of faculty from a nearby institution.

Benchmarking and best practices offer promise as adjuncts to the continuous improvement philosophy embedded in total quality management (TQM) programs. Use of quality improvement tools, coupled with the availability of appropriate data and the mind-set of continuous learning—a concept that the patient care executive must role model and vigorously support—will enhance clinician ability to investigate incremental improvement techniques that are often overlooked. Providing a supportive environment that empowers staff to take risks and ask significant clinical questions about traditional and accepted practices is fundamental to creative problem solving and productive clinical inquiry.

Conclusion

The patient care executive of the future must embrace and integrate the concept of stewardship with the traditional trappings of the role. *Stewardship* in this sense is broader than the traditional dictionary definition, which refers to a steward as one who supervises the provision and distribution of resources. In the greater context, stewardship is value driven and underpins decisions regarding the distribution and use of all resources, which is in line with the current emphasis on the business dimension of health care.

In the new health care culture, effective patient care executives must guide and support others to make the transition to the new environment and to operate effectively within it. This responsibility includes working to educate staff and managers, supporting clinical inquiry and creative problem solving, and supporting the use of research methodologies to add to the staff knowledge base. Thus, one dimension of the patient care executive's new role is to ensure that others are prepared to adjust the business of nursing.

References and Notes

1. The title *patient care executive* signifies the expanding role of the nurse executive. The responsibilities of the patient care executive often include oversight of the various departments that provide direct services to patients, including social work and pharmacy as well as nursing.

2. Burner, S., and Waldo, D. National health expenditure projections, 1994–2005. *Health Care Financing Review* 16(4):221, Summer 1995.

3. Russell, B. Opportunity costs in modern medicine. *Health Affairs* 11:162, Summer 1992.

4. Jameton, A. *Nursing Practice: The Ethical Issues.* Englewood Cliffs, NJ: Prentice-Hall, 1984.

Bibliography

Block, P. *Stewardship.* San Francisco: Barrett-Koehler, 1993.

Jameton, A. *Nursing Practice: The Ethical Issues.* Englewood Cliffs, NJ: Prentice-Hall, 1984.

Chapter 2

Seizing Opportunities in the New Health Care Delivery System

Richard Brock, MA, CNAA, RN

Over the years, nursing has demonstrated the ability to adapt to changes in health care practice and delivery, regardless of setting. One needs only to look at some of the recent monumental changes that have occurred in the switch from a system that rewarded manual dexterity in team nursing to one that rewards *cognitive nurses* (nurses who use critical thinking skills to provide new approaches to solving patient care problems) who are good at delivering primary care. Today, nursing is not only faced with cultural and attitudinal change, it is being repackaged to adapt to new care delivery systems such as case management and managed care. Nurses need to view these new systems as opportunities to use their unique knowledge and skills in the development of new approaches to patient care.

This chapter examines some of the shifts in thinking that nurses must make in order to adapt to the notion of health care as a business. It also clarifies some of the skills and behaviors that will facilitate that transition.

The Repackaging of Health Care Services

The notion of "packaging" or "repackaging" health care services is a business technique. That health care is a business as well as a service is evidenced by the naming, pricing, and marketing of specific services and procedures. In addition, the fact that Hospital X offers open-heart surgery and is located two blocks away from a potential patient who requires open-heart surgery is not a guarantee that *that* patient will choose Hospital X for his surgery. Patients are as sophisticated in making health care choices as they are in making choices about purchasing an automobile. They read *Consumer Reports* and select products based on quality, affordability, and a track record of customer satisfaction.

Within health care, decisions as to what to package and how are now made at management roundtables. Thus, the business of nursing has moved to the roundtable, where strategies for surviving and thriving are examined and determined. In reality, nurses may be the only participants at the "table" with clinical knowledge, which gives them a unique and important edge in determining the future of the business. To be successful in today's practice and to be effective roundtable participants, nurses must shift mental gears and develop new competencies.

Shifts in Thinking

In the coming years, nurses must forget some of the old paradigms and shape new ones. (See table 2-1.) Following are four examples of shifts in thinking that need to be in the nurse's survival kit. In the new forms of health care delivery, the successful nurse will need to:

1. Deliver care at the lowest reasonable price.
2. Provide the best experience for the patient and his or her family. Providing the best experience encompasses the processes of admission, treatment, and discharge from the hospital and includes posthospitalization follow-up. Customer service, marketing, and organizational survival are all directly related to providing the best experience.
3. Offer and develop a track record of excellent patient outcomes.
4. Focus on customer services with the same intensity and purpose that any successful business uses.

Competition is part of the new business culture in health care institutions. The hospital that succeeds is the one that can deliver what the customer needs and demands. Thus, as in any business, it is the customer who

Table 2-1. Old versus New Nursing Paradigms

Old Paradigm	New Paradigm
Success is based on high hospital census.	Payer mix is more important than patient census.
Nurses are rewarded for working double shifts.	Nurses are rewarded for cognitive and critical thinking skills to achieve outcomes.
FTEs are controlled to meet financial goals.	Cost per unit of service is controlled to meet goals.
Focus is on sick care and treatment.	Focus is on customer service.
Focus is on hospital care.	Focus is on caring for the patient in the right setting at the right time.

defines quality. In today's health care environment, quality as defined by the customer is a marketing tool and has business implications at every level of the organization. If health care organization CEOs and nursing administrators could view the business of the organization through the eyes of the customer, questions involving decisions related to hospital decor, signage, noise control, food, and general environmental ambience would be answered. Viewing the organization from the patient's point of view has implications for everyone in the organization, from admitting clerks to people in the business office, environmental services, and security to the bedside nurse.

The effective nurse executive will understand the business environment and what needs to be done from a clinical–economic–administrative–customer perspective. In this regard, he or she is a member of the management team and works with others in the institution's effort to achieve cost and quality outcomes. Because the relationship between nursing and the other disciplines on the management team (for example, physicians, financial officers, and administrators) is vital to the success, and indeed the survival, of the institution's care delivery system, relationship building is key among the new skills that nurses must acquire.

Shifts in Skills and Personal Approaches

Personal development is necessary to enhance any individual's talents. This is certainly true in the health care industry, where the ability to exert a positive influence is key to personal success. It is important to realize that the current crisis in health care is a result of how we are presently thinking. Thus, personal approaches and skills must be shifted just as the paradigms mentioned earlier must be. Important new skills and cues for key behaviors include:

- *Repositioning skills:* The nursing unit is being replaced by the patient care unit; respond to that fact enthusiastically. Invite communication from and with other health care disciplines that affect patient care delivery.

   In addition to clinical knowledge, be able to articulate an understanding of finance, human resource utilization, politics, and customer service. For example, demonstrate that services provided on the patient care unit are associated with the costs of the care encounter, staffing, interpersonal relationships, and service effectiveness.

- *Networking skills:* Do not try to reinvent the wheel; begin professional benchmarking with colleagues to learn about new practices and what works for them. For example, ask a social worker about child-care options for a patient who will be immobile after discharge from the hospital, or query an occupational therapist about interventions and devices that could help a stroke victim regain manual dexterity while in the hospital. In turn, share your innovations and successes.

- *Critical thinking skills:* Challenge systems and practices that have become nonproductive. It is important to revisit everything you think and do. If a particular long-standing practice does not add value, modify or even remove it. When viewed as a business, health care cannot afford to retain past practices that no longer work but are kept simply because they are familiar. For example, eliminating the unnecessary moving of patients from unit to unit keeps patients in familiar surroundings, prevents the loss of get-well cards, and avoids administrative confusion in the computer system. Additionally, reward staff for critical thinking and the ability to view changes as possibilities rather than roadblocks.
- *Risk-taking skills:* Examine the risks of risk taking. What is the worst that could happen if you dare act on a gut feeling or a new idea? Let comfort serve as a danger signal. In the learning curve, compile a "what I am going to do today" list and a "what I am not going to do today" list. For example, one might consider the risk of moving admissions to the patient care unit.
- *Skills for anticipating customer service needs:* Go shopping at businesses within the community that are known for high-quality customer service. Once you have experienced what customer service is all about from the customer's point of view, look at your hospital or health system as though you had never seen it before. What would make sense for the customer? What would the customer really value? For example, some customer service–oriented department stores' representatives actually shop for you based on a list you bring to them, and then they gift-wrap your purchases. Consider how such treatment might correspond to patient care; perhaps health care organizations should bring services to patients instead of transporting patients to services.

The reason for developing all of these appropriate behaviors is to influence the quality of patient care in its new forms.

Conclusion

Health care has a new form. In addition to providing opportunities for new experiences, the new form of health care is making challenging demands on nursing. As hospitals, physicians, trustees, and payer groups refocus to form alliances and networks to capture and maximize market share, they have only to ask customers what they want, what quality means to them, and how much they are willing to pay for it. Generally, the consumers of health care prefer to be treated in familiar surroundings such as the home, which has vast implications for the hospital as it is currently known. Nurse managers must be innovative, keeping options and opportunities for care beyond the hospital walls both in sight and in reach for customers. In the new form of health care, the savvy nurse must be thoughtful, innovative, willing to learn, and open to communication.

Chapter 3

Assessing the Cost-Effectiveness of Home Care

Katherine R. Jones, PhD, RN, FAAN

As discussed in earlier chapters, home health care and care delivered in other nonacute settings are increasingly viewed as lower-cost alternatives to hospital and nursing home care. However, to date, the evidence supporting this belief is mixed. Given that the expenditures for home health care delivery are increasing at a far more rapid rate than those for other categories of health care services, it is important to identify ways by which this care can be delivered in the most cost-effective manner possible. This is particularly important for nurse executives because the extension of care delivery into settings other than the hospital has placed new demands and expectations on the role and responsibilities of nurses.

This chapter illustrates the kind of data that nurse executives and other health care professionals will need to consider and evaluate in making decisions about care delivery in settings outside the hospital. It also describes some of the strategies being followed to improve the cost-effectiveness of providing care in these settings. Finally, this chapter concludes with a summary of implications for nurse executives in the new business environment.

Growth in Home Health Care Spending

Home health care is the fastest-growing component of Medicare expenditures, with Medicare spending on the home health benefit growing from $2.12 billion in 1988 to $10.5 billion in 1993.[1] Medicare home health expenditures have experienced annual growth rates exceeding 25 percent every year since 1988, and such expenditures consumed 5.3 percent of total Medicare spending in 1993.[2] Home health care spending has also increased significantly in the Medicaid program. Medicaid home health expenditures rose from $2 billion in 1988 to $4.5 billion in 1993.[3] Perhaps even more noteworthy is the increase associated with home- and community-based care waiver dollars, which grew from $3.8 million in 1982 to close to $3 billion in 1993.[4]

The characteristics of the growth in Medicare spending are of even more interest. Between 1988 and 1991, the charges per home care visit increased by 4.7 percent, less than the increase in the consumer price index and less than the increase in the Health Care Financing Administration market basket for home health input prices.[5] The number of Medicare beneficiaries receiving home health care services increased by 9 percent, with more than 6 percent of Medicare beneficiaries receiving home care in 1991.[6] The greatest growth has been in the number of home visits per beneficiary. In 1988, the average was 24.0; by 1991, it had risen to 44.5.[7] Little is known about the needs of these patients, for example, the duration, intensity, and mix of services required by these high-use beneficiaries. A 1990 study by Williams and others was able to explain only 4 to 11 percent of the variation in resource use per home care patient using payer status, prognosis, medical diagnosis, age, and hospital length of stay as predictor variables.[8] Two questions must be asked:

1. Will this growth in expenditures plateau, or will it continue to expand for years to come?
2. Should we be concerned about these home health care spending increases, or are they serving to reduce health care expenditures in other segments of the system and/or to produce higher-quality patient care outcomes?

The results of multiple research studies and demonstration projects have produced contradictory answers to the latter question.

Research and Demonstration Project Findings

Research studies and demonstration projects can be divided into two groups: those that focus on the elderly and those that focus on the nonelderly populations. The years of research on whether home health care is a cost-effective alternative to institutional care (primarily long-term care) have produced mixed results. They show that home care increased patient and informal caregiver satisfaction, reduced the number of unmet needs, and produced small gains in cognitive status; but they also raised overall health care expenditures, had no impact on activities of daily living, and had minimal impact on hospital use or nursing home admissions or days.[9] A meta-analysis of 13 studies concluded that home care had a small beneficial effect on mortality but a stronger positive effect on nursing home placements, reducing them by 23 percent.[10]

Studies within the Veterans Administration (VA) system also produced mixed results. The VA home care study, which focused on hospital-based home care versus routine care for chronically severely disabled patients, showed positive results for cognitive status and satisfaction of informal caregivers, as well as a 10 percent cost savings.[11] On the other hand, a VA adult day health care study found no differences between day-care and routine care groups in overall health status, psychological health, social health, or caregiver burden but an increase in patient satisfaction in the day-care group, with 15 percent higher costs in this group as well.[12]

Another study focused on care of patients with chronic obstructive pulmonary disease, randomizing these patients into one of three groups: standard office care, standard home health care, and specialized respiratory home care.[13] The study concluded that home care did not improve patient performance of daily activities, sense of general well-being, or pulmonary function, but did increase the total costs of care. Specialized home care was the most expensive; however, improved patient outcomes could not be detected.

Weissert, Cready, and Pawelak conducted a synthesis of 27 demonstration projects focused on home health care as a substitute for institutional care for the elderly. Their conclusions were that home care had not improved longevity, mental functioning, or physical functioning; nursing home use decreased slightly while life satisfaction improved slightly; and institutional cost savings were more than offset by increased use of home care.[14] Weissert recommended that policy analysts redirect their efforts to trying to make home health care more cost-effective by increasing savings on hospital or nursing home care, reducing the production costs of home care, and improving patient outcomes and thereby the value of the health status benefits.[15]

The Medicaid 2176 Home and Community-Based Waiver Program allows noninstitutional care for the aged, disabled, or mentally retarded. It primarily pays for case management, homemaker, personal care, and day-care services delivered to AIDS-infected adults and children, technology-dependent children, and nonelderly disabled adults. Again, the belief is that services delivered in noninstitutional settings will be more cost-effective, clinically appropriate, and preferred by patients, but supporting evidence is limited thus far.[16] Small-scale studies of technology-dependent children have suggested the following benefits: improvement in physical and physiologic functioning, reduced costs compared to inpatient care, strengthening of the family unit, and restoration of control of the child to the family.[17,18] However, these same studies suggested that home care of the technology-dependent child resulted in restriction of family activities, intrusion into family privacy, and a greater financial burden due to higher out-of-pocket costs. Aday and others concluded that creativity is needed to provide cost-effective alternatives to institutional care that reduce the rate of rehospitalization of these children while also reducing the level of stress experienced by the informal caregivers.[19]

Finally, positive results have been reported when using home visits as a mechanism to improve the outcomes of pregnancy and early child rearing among high-risk women.[20] These researchers were able to document a $1,664 net savings per family in government expenditures with the use of a nurse home visitor during pregnancy and for two years after the birth of the child. Other positive outcomes included reduced subsequent pregnancies, improved health-related behaviors, greater informal social support, and better use of the federal Women–Infant–Children's (WIC) Nutritional Program.

Strategies for Improving Cost-Effectiveness

It is extremely important that nursing and the home health industry focus on improving the documented cost-effectiveness of home health and other nonacute care services. Not to do so jeopardizes the continued funding of these services as well as limits the ability to argue for expanded funding for these types of programs. Several strategies can be pursued in this regard, many of which are relevant within integrated health care systems. These include:

- Shortening hospital stays
- Reducing hospitalization rates
- Reducing home health care costs
- Establishing a continuum of care

Shortening Hospital Stays

Hospital stays can be reduced through use of care coordination by case managers, which facilitates condition-specific early discharge. In addition, coordinated clinical pathways can be developed that include the inpatient, ambulatory, and home care services required by specific types of patients. These pathways would specify both the content and duration of home visits required by particular types of patients. Home infusion services can be provided for patients whose hospitalization is continued solely because of continuing antibiotic or nutritional support therapy requirements. Finally, telephone monitoring by ambulatory care nurses can be done for specific early-discharge patient groups, which has been shown to reduce the rate of rehospitalization among Medicare patients.

Reducing Hospitalization Rates

Strategies to reduce hospitalization rates of patients receiving home health care services include the use of physician home visits and direct-admission programs to long-term care settings or hospice care.[21] In addition, home infusion therapy can be utilized for groups that previously required hospitalization, such as for transplant rejection and chemotherapy.

Reducing Home Health Care Costs

The results of the studies previously reported in this chapter lead to several mechanisms by which the cost of home health care services may be reduced. One is to improve the screening of recipients, targeting those most likely to benefit from receipt of this type of service. These high-risk individuals include those who are older, mentally impaired, and functionally dependent. In addition, limits may need to be placed on the duration of services, based on the marginal benefits expected to be realized for continued visits to specific subgroups of recipients.[22] Some have recommended requiring regularly scheduled recertification of the need for home care services, with the process conducted by independent agencies. For example, in 1990, the Pepper Commission called for establishment of national practice guidelines for home care services.[23] More specifically, it would be helpful to develop home care pathways or protocols with predetermined time lines, expected outcomes, and specific interventions for subgroups of the home care population. Finally, various financial incentives may be put in place, including copayments and deductibles (perhaps based on a sliding scale) and bundled payments per episode of care, combining inpatient and home care service reimbursement.[24]

Establishing a Continuum of Care

Perhaps the most promising strategy to make home health care services, other nonacute care services, and institutional care more cost-effective is to establish a formal continuum of health care services. To do so would allow replacement of the current fragmented system with one that can facilitate placement of the recipient at the most appropriate level of care. This would allow reduced costs through more effective resource use and less waste. It also would facilitate achievement of other desired outcomes, including patient and caregiver satisfaction with services received and improvement in targeted patient clinical outcomes. An example is the St. Louis–based Carondelet Health Care System, which provides hospital-based home health services primarily for postdischarge acute care needs; case management for unstable acute and chronic patient care needs that transcend organizational boundaries; and community-based nursing care centers that focus on health promotion and maintenance, as well as disease prevention.[25]

Implications for Nurse Executives

Nurse executives can use several strategies to optimize the cost-effectiveness of subacute and postdischarge services delivered in the home. Referrals made for home health care services should be carefully considered. The practice of automatically referring specific types of patients to home care should be carefully scrutinized to ascertain whether the expected benefits exceed the costs of providing the additional service. Perhaps only those patients within a case-type who meet certain, specified criteria should receive a home health referral. A blanket system of referrals leads to wasted health care resources.

There should be specific, measurable clinical goals for each patient receiving home health care services. The number of home health visits made to any patient should be based on established treatment goals and not on the maximum number of visits allowed by reimbursement rules.

Careful coordination of home care services with inpatient care delivery creates the maximum benefit to the patient and the system. Early hospital discharge programs could be coordinated with structured home health care delivery programs. Specific types of patients could be managed along a clinical pathway that transcends organizational boundaries. The hospital would benefit from shorter hospital stays and lower readmission rates, and the home health care industry would benefit from a higher referral rate for subacute care services. Patients would also benefit by returning to the (usually) more desired home environment earlier, as well as from potentially lower rates of iatrogenic illnesses and nosocomial infections. Analyses should be performed to verify that overall costs to the health care system are lower through this coordinated care effort.

The nurse executive should actively support a clinical outcomes monitoring program. The components of such a program include both provider and patient assessments of the outcomes of care along the continuum of outcomes, ranging from complications to functional status to satisfaction. To achieve optimal patient care outcomes, it will be necessary to document and measure the content of care using a standardized nomenclature. Finally, the executive team should review all facets of care delivery to identify opportunities for new business ventures. Transitional care may present unique opportunities for development of new revenue streams. For example, a health care organization could consider establishing an infusion clinic, the primary service of which would be the training of patients and their primary caregivers in pump operation, dressing changes, and other aspects of self-care management related to home infusion therapy.

Conclusion

Home health and other nonacute care services probably will continue to grow at a rapid pace and will increasingly be viewed as an essential component of an integrated health care services delivery system. However, it is imperative that these services be delivered in the most cost-effective manner possible. Much more study is needed to identify the groups most likely to achieve benefits from such services, the outcomes that should be monitored and measured, and the organizational and system structures and processes that promote achievement of the desired outcomes.

References

1. Clauser, S. B. Recent innovations in home health care policy research. *Health Care Financing Review* 16(1):1–6, Fall 1994.

2. Clauser.

3. Clauser.

4. Clauser.

5. Bishop, C., and Skwara, K. C. Recent growth of Medicare home health. *Health Affairs* 12(3):95–110, Fall 1993.

6. Bishop and Skwara.

7. Bishop and Skwara.

8. Williams, B. C., Phillips, E. K., Torner, J. C., and Irvine, A. A. Predicting utilization of home health resources: important data from routinely collected information. *Medical Care* 28(5):379–91, May 1990.

9. Weissert, W. A new policy agenda for home care. *Health Affairs* 10(2):67–77, Summer 1991.

10. Hedrick, S. C., Koepsell, T. D., and Inui, T. Meta-analysis of home care effects on mortality and nursing home placement. *Medical Care* 27(11):1015–26, Nov. 1989.

11. Hughes, S. L., Cummings, J., Weaver, F., Manheim, L. M., Conrad, K. J., and Nash, K. A randomized trial of Veterans Administration home care for severely disabled veterans. *Medical Care* 28(2):135–45, Feb. 1990.

12. Rothman, M. L., Hedrick, S. C., Bulcroft, K. A., Erdly, W. W., and Nickinovich, D. G. Effects of VA adult day care on health outcomes and satisfaction with care. *Medical Care* 31(9):SS38–SS49, Sept. 1993.

13. Bergner, M., Hudson, L. D., Conrad, D. A., Patmont, C. M., McDonald, G. J., Perrin, E. B., and Gilson, B. S. The cost and efficacy of home care for patients with chronic lung disease. *Medical Care* 26(6):566–79, June 1988.

14. Weissert, W. G., Cready, C. M., and Pawelak, J. E. The past and future of home- and community-based long term care. *The Milbank Quarterly* 66(2):309–88, 1988.

15. Weissert.

16. Miller, N. A. Medicaid 2176 home and community-based waivers: the first ten years. *Health Affairs* 11(4):162–71, Winter 1992.

17. Burr, B. H., and others. Home care for children on respirators. *New England Journal of Medicine* 309(21):1319–23, Nov. 24, 1983.

18. Lawrence, P. A. Home care for ventilator-dependent children. *Dimensions of Critical Care Nursing* 3(1):42–52, Jan.–Feb. 1984.

19. Aday, L. A., Wegener, D. H., Anderson, R. M., and Aitken, M. J. Home care for ventilator-assisted children. *Health Affairs* 8(2):137–47, Summer 1989.

20. Olds, D. L., Henderson, C. R., Phelps, C., Kitzman, H., and Hanks, C. Effect of prenatal and infancy nurse home visitation on government spending. *Medical Care* 31(2):155–74, Feb. 1993.

21. Weissert.

22. Weissert.

23. The Pepper Commission. *A Call for Action. Final Report—U.S. Bipartisan Commission on Comprehensive Health Care.* Washington, DC: U.S. Government Printing Office, 1990.

24. Weissert.

25. Hey, M. Nursing's renaissance: an innovative continuum of care takes nurses back to their roots. *Health Progress* 74(8):26–32, Oct. 1993.

Chapter 4

Succeeding in a Market-Driven Environment: A Case Study

Julianne M. Morath, MS, RN

Abbott Northwestern Hospital, a large, tertiary care center located in Minneapolis, is typical of hospitals nationwide that are learning to provide care to patients and families in a market-driven environment. In the hospital's effort to apply a business mentality to its system of care delivery, its care providers, in particular, have had to overcome concerns over compromising professional values and standards.

This chapter focuses on the success of Abbott Northwestern's nursing department in making the transition to delivering care in a market-driven environment. In addition to describing the nursing department's journey, the chapter highlights some of the innovative programs that have resulted from the change process. An appendix at the back of the chapter condenses some of the requirements for practice in the new business environment.

The Movement of Business into Health Care: Background

In the past 10 years, employer demands, the move to capitation, and a significant reduction in the demand for certain health care services all have led to the development of large, integrated systems across the country, including in the Twin Cities and surrounding regions. Today, the health care market in the Twin Cities is characterized by:

The author would like to acknowledge these individuals for their spirit, expertise, and leadership: Mary Koloroutis; Carol Huttner; Ann Watkins; Ruth Sohl-Krieger; Pat Hartwig; Elaine Slocumb; Monica Sieg; Marjean Leary; Elaine Hogan-Miller; Phyllis Collier; Ginger Malone; Marge Watry; Terry Voigt; Audrey Haag; Robert K. Spinner; Todd Miller, MD; Sarah Horsman; Debra Waggoner; Deidre Perkins; and Nancy Garner Ebert. The author also would like to acknowledge the nurses, physicians, and employees at Abbott Northwestern Hospital for their work that created the content of this chapter.

- The alignment of insurers with providers, and physician practices with hospitals
- An increased number of physician group practices, physician–hospital organizations, and system-owned practices
- Increased opportunities for providers such as nurse practitioners, wellness and health specialists, and chiropractors, among others
- Increased cooperation in the area of technology among institutions
- The issue of excess hospital bed capacity

As a result, in their attempts to provide care, health care institutions in the Twin Cities are faced with:

- Continued provider integration and shrinkage in the inpatient market
- More and stronger competition for inpatient care and specialty referrals
- Greater accountability for the community's health
- Increased system emphasis on clinical integration and efficiency
- Larger and more assertive buyer coalitions
- Continued focus on primary care as the center of health care delivery
- Continued proliferation of technology at a time when rationalization and regionalization have become survival strategies
- Stagnating federal and state health reform (although the reform of integrated delivery systems continues to progress)

The purchasers of health care are clear about their needs: predictable, stable, affordable prices; elimination of what they perceive as unnecessary and inappropriate care; a network of convenient primary care and specialty providers; and data to support continued value improvement in health care, especially in outcome research.[1]

Making the transition from a patient-driven to a market-driven health care system requires hospitals to make significant shifts in thinking and to acquire a business orientation. It requires that hospitals move from knowing what they think is best for their customers to learning what their customers require of them. It requires care providers to shift from making decisions independently to making decisions interdependently. This new business orientation means moving beyond relying on routines, rituals, and individual preferences to providing data-based care and searching for the best practice, from complex system messes to simplified processes and systems that fulfill customer needs; from giving everything to the patient to providing the patient with the best value (defined as the best cost and quality outcome), with service quality as the distinguishing advantage.

The movement of business into health care has produced integrated networks that align the incentives and services of providers, delivery systems, and health plans into a single organization. Their combined focus is on cost reduction, process improvement, and value creation. The integrated service network model first surfaced in 1962 when Alfred Dupont Chandler, historian of business at the Harvard Business School, suggested that when manufacturing systems were integrated, the resulting cost and service advantages would enable those businesses to dominate their industry.[2]

In the health care industry, similar realignments will satisfy a number of purposes, including:

- Creating an integrated system
- Accepting a single check from a public or private sponsor for an enrolled population
- Using the resulting pool of funds to cover the health needs of that population
- Ensuring that everyone involved in the care of that population gets paid

All this, it is believed, will be easier to do if the pieces of the system are integrated and owned or employed by a single organization. Does this type of integration work in health care? The jury is still out.[3]

The Transition at Abbott Northwestern Hospital

At Abbott Northwestern Hospital, the transition to a stronger business orientation is well under way. The hospital is now part of Allina, an integrated service network whose name connotes alignment. Allina brings together providers, delivery sites, and insurance products. As part of an integrated service network, the system's measure of success is changing from *patients* to *covered lives*. Hospitals are viewed as expense centers, and their use of resources must be contained or reduced. In the new system, the site of care is increasingly being relocated to home, community, nursing home, school, and other less-intensive, less-invasive settings. (Futurists predict that within this decade, 80 percent of the procedures currently being performed in hospital main operating rooms will be relocated to outpatient settings.) Abbott Northwestern's licensed capacity of 900 beds was often full. Today, the operating capacity is 500 beds with a fluctuating census. Length of stay (LOS) is 5.2 days, and intensity of care is increasing steadily.

Care Documentation

As the hospital moves toward a stronger business orientation, employers are requiring documentation of the plan to organize, sequence, and deliver care and services for case types—a *care pathway* or documented process of care. The business world has used process identification and measurement since Walter Shewhart of Bell Laboratories introduced the concept of the control chart, a simple but powerful tool of business measurement.[4] Today, health care organizations are beginning to identify care processes and key organizational or support processes and place them in control. Historically, health care organizations have been organized around departments or professions as they serve patients. The identification of processes across traditional boundaries and points of disconnection provides the opportunity for integration that will eliminate duplication, competition, and fragmentation.

At Abbott Northwestern, the key processes identified in the plan for patient care are:

- Wellness and prevention
- Assessment and diagnosis
- Intervention and therapy
- Caring and relating

The last process in the preceding list reflects the personal and therapeutic dimensions of the relationships involved in health care. Support processes include accessing, planning, documenting, coordinating, information processing, educating, resource allocating, and monitoring.[5] (See figure 4-1.)

The Documentation Tool

In nursing care delivery, the primary documentation tool is the care pathway, which stabilizes and documents the process of care by diagnosis-related group (DRG), reflecting the interdisciplinary collaboration required to implement care for a defined population. *Care pathways* are the clinical processes — the specific practices in the delivery of patient care for a specific case type — that guide the sequencing, coordination, and detailing of specific elements of the care process. They are used to track costs and identify trends. When these care processes are stabilized, they can be measured and improved. The compression of variance and identification of best practice is a focus.

In the acute care setting, a variance committee measures deviation from the expected pathway. (*Variance* is the measure of deviation between what happened and what was expected to happen during a patient's care.) This measure provides meaningful information that can be used to evaluate the care processes and identify improvement opportunities. Variance studies focus on the key events identified by a multidisciplinary team during pathway design. The variance data can be used to improve the care of a specific patient to either continually advance his or her progress or reassess the plan for care.

Variance from a pathway also can be analyzed for a group of patients, and a pathway thus becomes a tool that supports quality improvement and outcome measurement. A pathway variance study begins by focusing the patient population. The principle of *leverage,* or determining where the greatest impact can be made, is used. Things to consider when determining the patient population include the top DRG list, quality reports, satisfaction

Figure 4-1. Patient Care Delivery Model

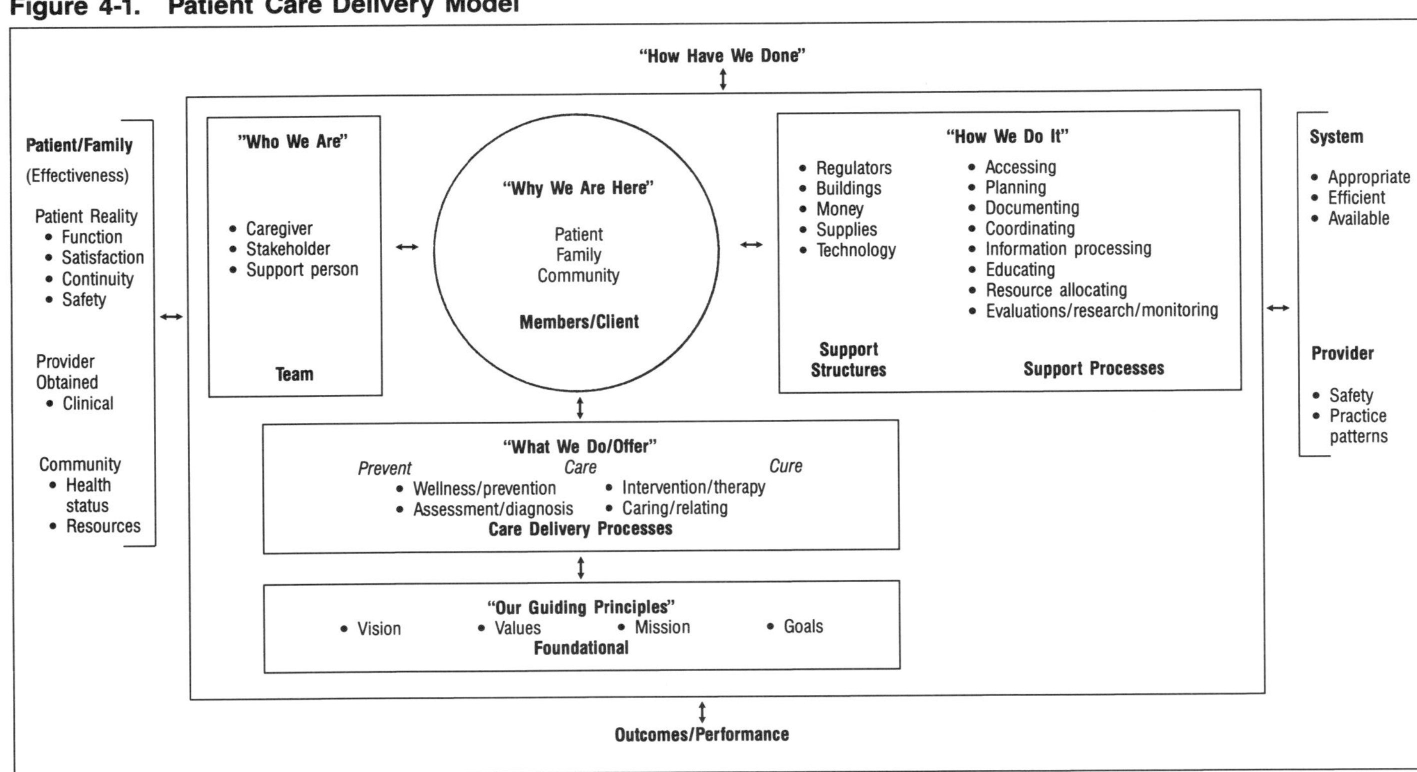

surveys, populations at risk, outcome management strategies, or studies in process. The study team determines the sample size and time frame needed to collect the data. Data collection can be done through concurrent input of data or retrospective review. Data are analyzed by a variety of possible resources, including pathway development groups, patient care councils, quality management staff, and those involved in continuous quality improvement (CQI) projects. Findings are communicated, and plans for improvement are made by identifying the potential explanations for the identified variance. Assessment is made as to whether the explanation was valid, findings are documented, data are analyzed, and interventions are made by modifying or changing the process of care. Finally, the variance study efforts are evaluated, and the need for further study to evaluate the effectiveness of the intervention is identified.

Following are examples of how pathway variance studies were used at Abbott Northwestern and their results:

- One study undertaken by the neuroscience division to evaluate the microdiscectomy pathway showed that 83 percent of patients had a variance in pain management. A multidisciplinary team consisting of neurosurgeons, nurses, and a pharmacist analyzed medication-specific data and other pain interventions for these patients. Based on data from the analysis, the team incorporated Agency for Health Care Policy and Research (AHCPR) guidelines on acute pain management into the pathway, including generic postoperative orders. Follow-up variance data have shown that only 19 percent of patients now have pain as a variance, an improvement of 64 percent. The reduction in variance has resulted in improved patient care, reduced LOS, and reduced charges.[6]
- With bypass surgery patients reporting that the single worst aspect of their procedure was having the endotracheal tube in so long after surgery, the bypass surgery value enhancement team decided to draft clinical criteria for tube removal. The result was that in only three years, early extubation increased from just 2 to 58 percent. Not only can patients now move more freely and communicate with their families, but there has been a decrease in infection rate, a reduction in the amount of sedation required, and a full-day reduction in LOS in the intensive care unit.

The hospital now is in the process of attaching supply utilization to the care pathway with the intention of isolating and measuring resources and costs. It is conceivable that this could lead to a preferred supplier system in which a supplier with a demonstrable quality program, best cost, and willingness to enter into a long-term relationship and share risk in capitation is selected to work exclusively with the hospital. This requires measurement and joint monitoring of utilization, quality, and cost trends.

The Impact of Business Science on the Art of Caring

When considering how business science will affect care delivery, one question that arises is: Can the processes of care truly be standardized? Unlike the manufacturing process, variability in the human response to illness creates variability in individual expressions of disease. For example, people may express their illnesses and respond to interventions in markedly distinctive ways based on their level of knowledge about their illness, their history, their level of anxiety, and the presence or absence of a support system.

The relationship between members of the clinical community and patients/families is unique and based on individualized requirements. As patients/families become the clinical community's partners in care, the hospital's ability to execute the process of care to meet the unique requirements of the individual will be the distinguishing advantage for providers and organizations. This is thought of as management of the patient/family experience of care.

A reductionistic and mechanistic application of business science in health care without use of the art of caring can be limiting. The danger exists that this would diminish the caring and relating processes of the hospital's work. At the center of this work is an intentional caring that creates the safety necessary for healing, empowerment, and growth. This caring is intimate and personal, and is not expressed in a case-specific care pathway or process.

Can discipline be applied to this intentional caring? The answer is yes, through the measurement of sentient quality. *Quality,* a word that is read, spoken, and heard daily in health care today, has two dimensions of emphasis. These are best defined in Gerteis's book *Through the Patient's Eyes,* which describes the Picker-Commonwealth study of patient satisfaction.[7]

One dimension has to do with technical excellence. This includes professional skill and competence, and the capacity of diagnostic and therapeutic equipment, procedures, and systems to accomplish what they are meant to accomplish reliably and effectively in a way that is readily measurable and quantifiable.

The second dimension is more difficult to measure but cannot be diminished or ignored. It relates to the texture and substance of personal experience, and sometimes is referred to as *sentient quality*—the quality of a sensation and experience or the quality of a human relationship. It is in this dimension of caring that true healing occurs, because it is this dimension that patients/families experience most directly. Gerteis aptly describes how this dimension influences patient/family perceptions of safety and well-being, responses to illness, and feelings of receiving care. Patients/families develop these perceptions through interactions with professional providers, observations of providers' interactions with each other, and experiences in the settings in which services are provided.

Today, health care providers face unyielding issues of access, cost, and clinical effectiveness. Especially now, they must be ever aware of the experiential dimension of their practice. Providers know that patients want and need an enhanced sense of well-being that incorporates respect, choice, privacy, safety, and relief from the effects of illness. A therapeutic relationship, no matter how brief, affords the opportunity for true caring and healing to take place, thus allowing the artistry and the science of health care to be practiced simultaneously to achieve quality of care.

Some aspects of the patient/customer requirements described in the Picker-Commonwealth study can be met through deliberate, disciplined approaches to care and by placing a process in control, such as systematic implementation of AHCPR pain guidelines. However, other aspects of care, such as respect, depend on the quality of relationships established among unique individuals based on assessment of need and understanding of the caring phenomenon.

Is the use of business systems diminishing the care provided to patients? Today, patients are asking more from hospitals than they have been given previously. For example, they are asking for cost and quality outcomes. They are requiring seamless, integrated care that is communicated to them clearly and in which they can participate. And they are requiring access to service and service quality. Responding to customer requirements is both good business and good care.

References to business systems often highlight only the production model of business. This focus does not recognize that around half of today's business systems produce services. Business consists of both service and production. Hospitals, clinics, and other health care organizations have much in common with service business models. For example, practices related to the hotel industry and business concepts such as expectation theory and purchase behavior clearly apply to the provision of health care services.

Making the transition to this market-driven environment in which business practices are used requires discipline, a grounding in professional practice that includes the patient/customer as a participant, and an organizational context to support the work. This begins with an intentional and systemic approach to change. The remainder of this chapter highlights the foundational work for that change in Abbott Northwestern Hospital's nursing department.

The Nursing Department's Journey of Change

Abbott Northwestern Hospital has been an engine of growth and financial success throughout its history. It was process oriented, with less emphasis on outcome. Its structure was decentralized with a traditional hierarchy that focused on discrete functional areas and multiple systems and processes that operated independently. This was not sustainable. Following is a description of how the transition to a market-driven mentality was accomplished within the hospital's nursing department.

Building the Vision

The nursing department's journey of change began firmly grounded in philosophy and vision. The department's philosophy was retested to act as a moral compass through the change process. It is based on advocacy through caring. The department's vision represents the shared vision of more than 300 nurses, each with a personal view of the ideal practice experience.

Personal visions were elicited from three sources:

1. Nurses who attended educational sessions entitled Advocacy through Caring
2. Nurses who attended retreats entitled Personal Mastery
3. Participants from ongoing focus groups with the nurse executive

The resultant vision was simple and powerful:

Patients are the reason we exist. People are the reason we excel. Systems support the work.

The complete vision is provided in figure 4-2.

Assessing the Current Reality

An assessment of the current reality of nursing practice was conducted using the same three sources that helped build the department's vision, and a

Figure 4-2. The Vision of the Nursing Department, Abbott Northwestern Hospital

Practice—Patients are the reason we exist.

The philosophy of nursing is lived in practice every day by each nurse. Nurses practice their profession with confidence, compassion, and skill.

Relationships—People are the reason we excel.

Through our words and actions, nurses inspire, recognize, and reward leadership and expect care for the caregiver; and require professional development and collaborative governance.

Diversity in nursing is our strength. Our ability to collaborate brings our best to the patient and strengthens our profession. This strength and energy allow us to enter into collegial relationships that produce extraordinary results on behalf of our patients and the organization.

Systems—Systems support the work.

Nurses are wise stewards of resources and use the tools, methods, and technology of quality improvement and innovation to refine practice and influence the systems that affect it.

systematic inventory of the system of care delivery was conducted by the department's nurse leaders. The assessment resulted in a painful but candid reflection of the gap between vision and reality. This gap provided the energy for change.

A specific plan of operations was established to move the nursing organization toward its new vision. To show that patients were the reason the department existed, the plan recognized the need to identify patient-focused customer requirements. To show that people were the reason the department excelled, operational goals included creation of an informed, competent workforce with access to the necessary skills and support to learn and develop continuously. To create systems that supported the work, the plan reflected the department's aim to reduce complexity, identify and improve key processes, and redesign work and access to information. The plan focused the department's priorities and moved it toward outcome orientation.

More specifically, the three parts of the vision were embodied in the daily work of the nursing department in various ways. To develop the *patients are the reason we exist* part of the vision statement, the department focused on improving its ability to listen to customers. Patient surveys, focus groups, and patient participation in care delivery redesign were used to increase the department's knowledge of patient requirements and perceptions, and data resulting from these initiatives were used to create action plans to improve customer service and nurse responsiveness. Today, whenever tensions arise concerning a course of action, the question "What would the patient expect of us in this situation?" is used to consider and resolve the issue. The Personal Mastery retreat (described later in this chapter), a program to increase the capacity of employees to contribute to the success of the organization, was established to embody the value *people are the reason we excel. Systems support the work,* the third component of the vision, has been evidenced through the support of process improvement teams working on issues such as improving case cart completion in the operating room, simplifying and improving the patient registration process, and implementing a point-of-care computerized clinical documentation system for the intensive care unit.

Building a Supportive Structure

A new structure was needed to release the collective talent and intellect of the nursing department so that it could move toward its new vision. The first reorganization resulted in the notion of a matrix to (1) identify key processes that would provide an infrastructure to support, rather than direct, the work of nursing and patient care and (2) assign accountability for those processes. As figure 4-3 shows, the vertical axis represented program/operational responsibilities, and the horizontal axis introduced the emphasis on key processes that crossed all operational areas. These processes

Figure 4-3. Infrastructure Matrix That Supports the Work of Nursing at Abbott Northwestern Hospital

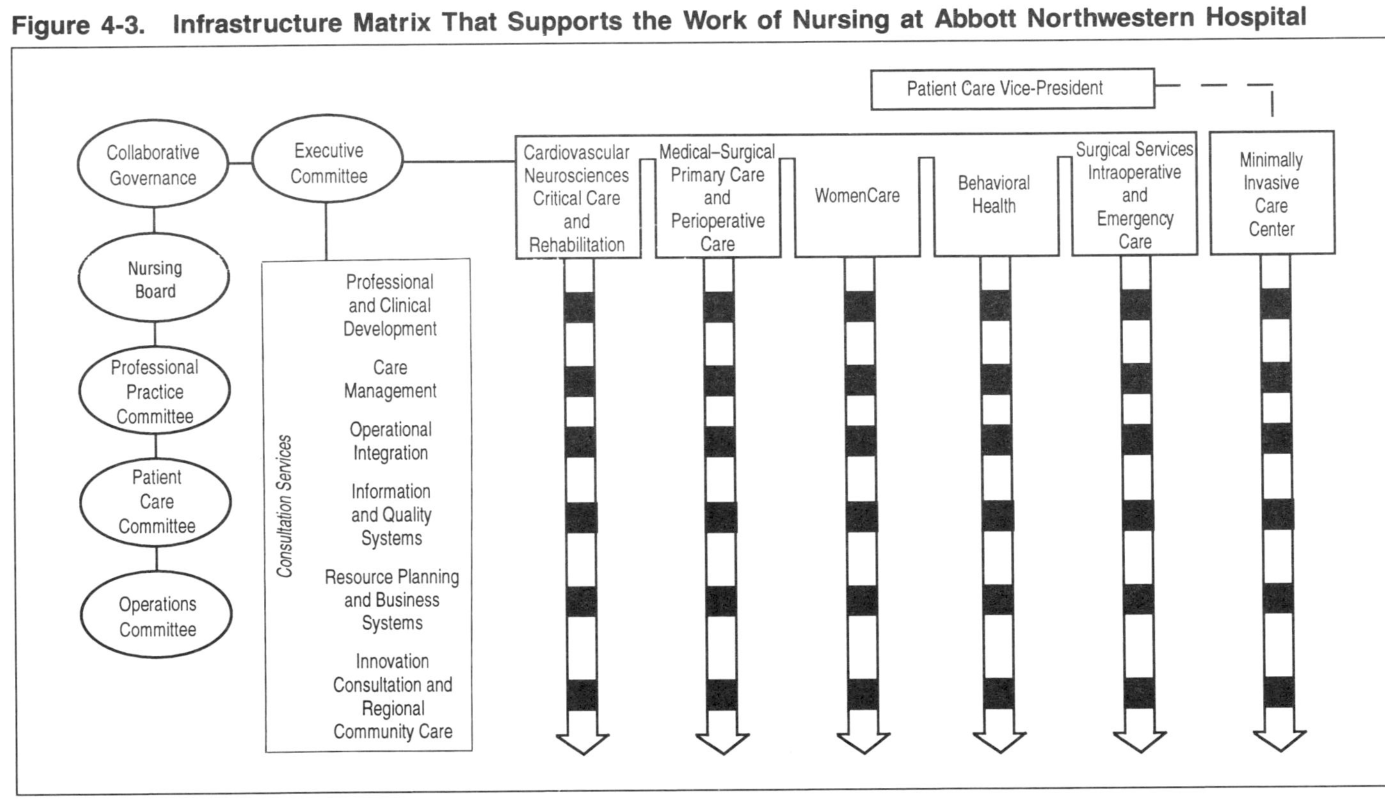

Source: Used with permission of Abbott Northwestern Hospital, Minneapolis.

included professional and clinical development; care management; operational integration or assurance of coordination across division boundaries; information and quality systems; resource planning and business systems; and innovation, consultation, and regional community care.

The structure was designed to support the functional areas and also to identify, strengthen, and manage the department's key processes—the infrastructure or foundation upon which care is delivered. Its intent was to create a leaner, more horizontal organization. The structure recognized the ability of nurses to be full partners in the governance of practice. It created an interdependence among nursing leaders, and the focus and alignment to end internal competition and duplication and to enhance collaboration. Its focus was on patients and care processes rather than on the departments and divisions in which care was delivered. This structure is reflected in the nursing department's collaborative governance structure, now four years old. An operations plan reflects the department's intention, and an implementation plan reflects its commitment to achieve its vision. Priorities for action and resources are established by the operations plan.

The nursing department structure had clear guiding principles:

- The department is integrating and aligning to support high-quality patient care.
- The structure is not hierarchical; nurses will function as a team for the benefit of the whole department.
- The structure supports department priorities to focus nursing's activities with an emphasis on outcomes.
- The structure is based on the principles of a learning organization, capitalizing on the collective strengths and talents of all members rather than on the skills of individual members.
- Communication will be key to the department's success. This includes not only communication between nurses but also between the nursing department and its various constituencies about what is and is not working.
- Concerns about changes will be discussed openly. If withheld, they will likely come out when it is too late to make a difference.
- Nurses cannot work as a team unless they are a team. This will necessitate a commitment of time, energy, and expertise.
- Nurses must be clear about the expected outcomes and be willing to set their course to achieve them.
- The vision must be clearly articulated and must include priorities.

The nurse director role was retitled nurse leader/consultant, and its responsibilities shifted from those of an advocate for a given department to those of a leader who would:

- Ensure the integration and alignment of the pieces to the whole organization

- Develop and implement strategic direction by engaging in strategic dialogue, by being the steward of the organization's resources, and by being the hospital's eyes and ears in anticipating change
- Create, lead, perpetuate, and sustain a shared vision, values, and culture
- Be a living example of quality principles such as mentoring, teaching, and stewardship
- Ensure that the organization has effective systems by identifying and validating them, devoting resources to their success, and evaluating them by determining whether they had a broad impact, were cost-effective, and facilitated achievement of intended outcomes
- Communicate with, be a resource for, consult with, and partner with others and the organization to solve problems
- Understand and respond to customer requirements and perceptions

Creating Communities of Care

The combined pressures of declining inpatient census and rising costs required greater flexibility and more facile movement of staffing and beds to meet changing requirements, which included census fluctuations as great as 20 percent in either direction within patient care units and the fact that distribution of patient population by specialty varied greatly. At the same time, the need for highly competent staff who were able to advance the plan of care was essential.

This dilemma led to the creation of communities of care. These patient-centered communities among units that share common elements gave staff and managers more flexibility in responding to changing requirements. The reorganization reduced management positions, improved relationships among patient care areas, built new partnerships, and reflected changes made by nurses through the collaborative governance process. Issues of "being pulled" or "floating" to another unit diminished as territories became less demarcated. Nurses were able to be more versatile in their practice. The communities of care created a new sense of "us," rather than the culture of "we and they" that sometimes exists between specialties. Examples of communities are medical–surgical care, cardiovascular care, orthoneuroscience–rehabilitative care, and WomenCare.

The word *community* was chosen carefully and deliberately, and was influenced by the work of Dr. M. Scott Peck.[8] It connotes a group of people committed to a common purpose and to each other. The notion of community transforms the interaction between nurse and hospital from a purely financial transaction (where the nurse's skills are purchased to complete work) to a collaborative effort in which both nurse and hospital serve a common purpose.

Within communities of care, nurse managers partner with each other in the provision of leadership, each with a different yet complementary focus.

These partnerships are formed of tough, compassionate, complementary-skilled managers committed to common goals. Peter Senge suggests that the essential component of a learning organization is the learning partnership two people can form when they are communicating and working together.[9] Such a partnership is unique and provides structure. Each individual brings to it a new way of interacting and feeling that facilitates commitment. It improves the quality of thinking and decision making, and models the essentials of learning for the community, councils, and work groups.

The partnership encourages managers to rid themselves of traditional approaches to managing or leading other people and to move toward empowerment and facilitation. They have not job-shared but have analyzed and distributed the work to become more effective. A computer local-area network system has created virtual centralization that gives access to real-time data to support decision making, information sharing, and learning.

The Results of the Journey

Over the course of two years, the nursing department's organizational structure matured to look like the model shown in figure 4-4. This model represents how nursing practice now works within the organizational structure of the hospital. Its emphasis is on the relationship of the nurses' work—and the means by which it is accomplished—to patients, rather than on reporting relationships among individuals. In the model, the work of the nursing department is defined by the requirements of the patient populations it serves. The areas of nursing governance and practice; process pathways; and clinical practice model standards, guidelines, and protocols are the responsibility of the nursing practice division. For figure 4-4, the following areas are included under the umbrella of wellness–prevention, episodic care, acute–rehabilitative care, and maintenance and chronic care:

- Clinical nurse specialist group practice
- Enterstomal nursing
- Emergency care
- Healthy communities
- Outreach
- Consultation
- WomenCare
- Medical/surgical care
- Minimally invasive care center
- Ambulatory care
- Surgical services
- Perioperative care
- Critical care

Figure 4-4. Patient Care: Nursing Services Component

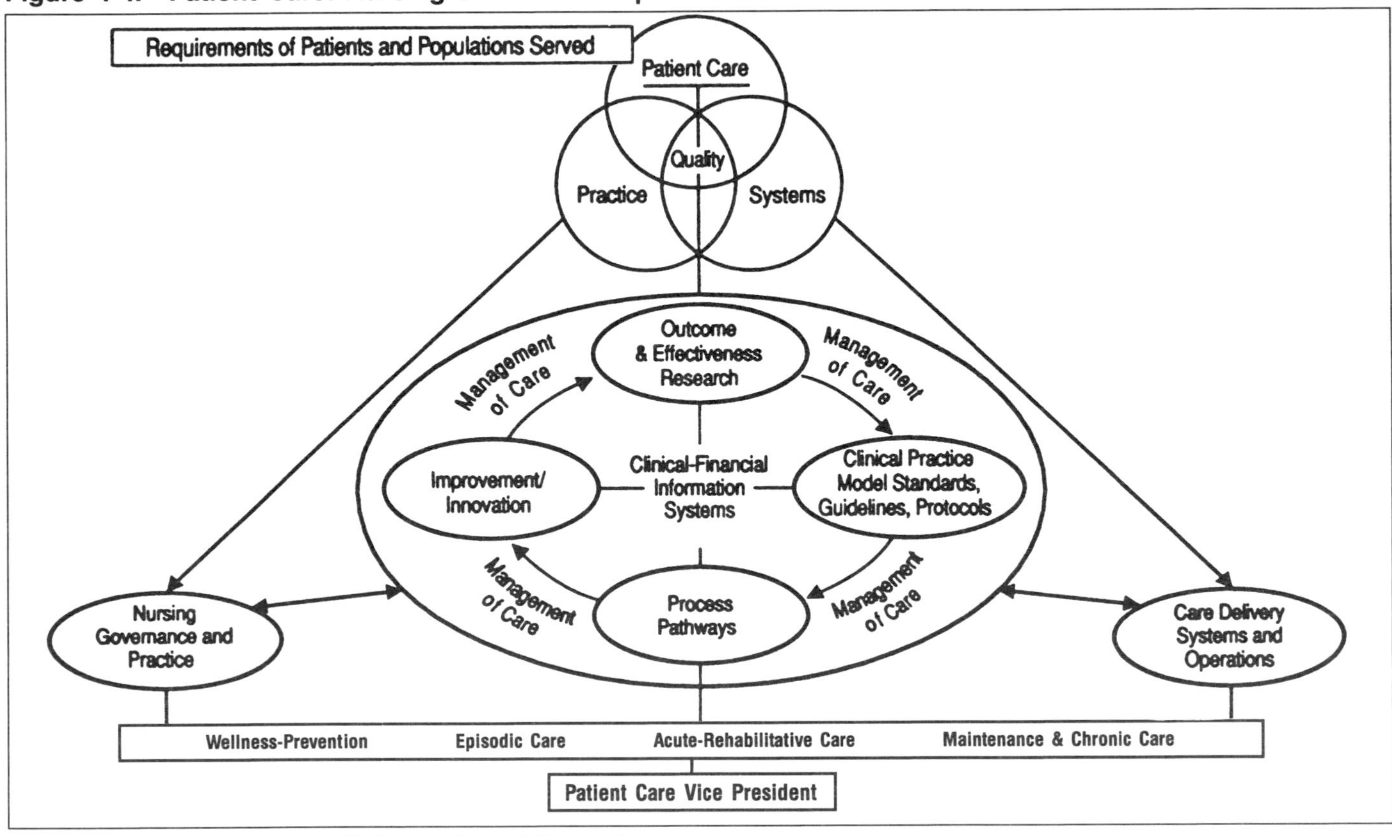

Source: Used with permission of Abbott Northwestern Hospital, Minneapolis.

- Cardiovascular–renal care
- Ortho–back–transitional care unit–neuro–rehab care
- Oncology
- Virginia Piper Cancer Institute care
- Behavioral health care

Three organizing principles—patient care, practice, and systems—described in the department's vision are used to structure the department's work:

1. *Patient care:* Patient care is the purpose of the department; in other words, it is the reason the department exists. Each member of the nursing department is responsible and accountable for patient care; this principle is the embodiment of nursing's philosophy and reflects its commitment to quality.

   Nursing care is data-based assessment, nursing diagnosis, planning, intervention, and evaluation of outcomes of care. Patient care requires that nursing care be integrated into the work of the care team, coordinating aspects of intervention and services required by patients/families across the continuum of care. The outcomes of patient care to be measured include patient, family, and community perception of function, health status, knowledge, safety, continuity, and satisfaction.

2. *Practice:* This is the domain that supports the work of patient care by ensuring that nurses and other direct or supportive caregivers and staff are appropriately licensed and that competencies based on standards of clinical practice are established, performances measured, competence ensured, and practice enhanced through continuing clinical and professional development. Practice outcomes to be measured include provider practice patterns, competency, safety, and meaningful work.

3. *Systems:* Systems include the methods, tools, procedures, and relationships that facilitate the work of patient care and integrate nursing into the whole of patient care delivery across the health care system. Patient flow, information transfer, communication, and cooperative relationships on a practical, daily basis depend on systems. Systems outcomes to be measured include the appropriateness, efficiency, and availability of resources.

The area of nursing governance and practice is the one in which the necessary nursing talent and expertise is coordinated to support practice capabilities and accountabilities. Care delivery systems and operations represent the coordination of leaders who support the systems of operations, resource allocation, and coordination and alignment of actions in the provision of patient care through the operations plan.

The Quality of Care Delivery

The principles of patient care, practice, and systems find integration through quality. *Quality* encompasses the mind-set, culture, theories, tools, and methods for continuously pursuing excellence that inspire vision and patient-focused care. In clinical nursing practice, quality is achieved through each individual's commitment to do the right thing, in the right way, at the right time, and in the right sequence to achieve reliable, predictable, and desired outcomes.

Quality also is each individual's willingness to work according to data-based standards, to be measured against those standards, and to be accountable for continuously improving performance. This work is achieved through:

- Use of the standards, guidelines, and protocols of the professional practice model
- Development and use of interdisciplinary pathways to guide the process of care
- Use of variance studies and other strategies to improve care and discover care innovations
- Use of research to add to nursing's knowledge and understanding of its work

The work of quality is supported through the collection, organization, integration, and analysis of clinical and financial data for decision making and learning.

The Continuum of Care Delivery

Care is provided according to care management strategies that recognize that there is a continuum in the patient experience that needs to be coordinated across delivery sites, geography, providers, services, and resources. Care and services are provided episodically in intervals from minutes to hours; in emergency, outpatient, minimally invasive care settings to acute, inpatient hospital settings; and over time in a variety of settings for maintenance, chronic, and hospice care. Increasingly, attention to wellness and prevention is emphasized in work with individuals, populations, and communities.

The Organization of Care Delivery

With attention to the continuum, the organization of care delivery is provided through the communities of care discussed earlier. Clinical nurse managers work in partnership to manage these communities and to provide practice leadership to achieve efficient and effective outcomes. Each community has a qualified nurse leader/consultant.

The administrative structure of the hospital is aligned so that the nurse leader/consultant works directly with administrators and physicians to plan, facilitate, evaluate, and enhance the program areas they represent. Nurse leaders/consultants have a direct, functional reporting relationship to the patient care vice-president (or to an operations vice-president), who is a qualified registered nurse executive, for professional standards of care and practice; for review of licensure and competence; and for access to consultation, decision making, care coordination, and educational and professional activities. The patient care vice-president provides clinical and administrative leadership and support, and is steward to the delivery of high-quality patient care and professional practice.

Innovations Supporting Organizational Change

Several key innovations made the restructuring of the nursing department possible. These included:

- The collaborative governance model
- The Advocacy through Caring program
- The Personal Mastery program

The Collaborative Governance Model

Collaborative governance is a communication and decision-making model that places the responsibility, authority, and accountability for nursing care with the practicing nurse. This is achieved through a clinical nursing structure that integrates with the management/administrative structure to create an environment of shared vision and excellence in patient care and nursing practice.

The model is implemented through a system of councils, committees, and a board, which have responsibility, accountability, and authority for conducting the business of the nursing department in the areas of strategic planning, development and evaluation, patient care, professional practice, and operational efficiency. The ongoing assessment of the functioning of collaborative governance is vital to its continued efficiency and effectiveness.

The collaborative governance model recognizes the knowledge, creativity, and talent of the clinical staff, and is recognized as a vehicle for bringing to daily practice the nursing philosophy and clinical practice model core beliefs.

The clinical structure of collaborative governance is based on these beliefs:

- Knowledge with participation is power.
- Given sufficient information, people will make appropriate decisions.

- Individuals are unique in their contributions.
- A sense of purpose, commitment, and optimal productivity results when organizational and personal goals are congruent.
- Risk taking, in itself, is growth.
- Differences are valued and offer the opportunity for learning.
- People are honest and trustworthy and will work hard to achieve their full potential.
- Individuals are accountable and responsible for their practice.
- Problems identified are mutually owned, and responsibility for resolution begins with problem identification.
- Collaboration with other departments and disciplines is essential to fulfill the hospital's mission.
- Individuals are empowered to meet their full potential.

The Advocacy through Caring Program

Advocacy through Caring is a major tenet of nursing department philosophy at Abbott Northwestern Hospital. The philosophy describes values and beliefs that are at the foundation of professional practice. The Advocacy through Caring program is planned for RNs during their first quarter of employment and for colleagues who want the opportunity to personalize and invest in the philosophy as it relates to their individual practice. Its content focuses on the nursing department's vision and direction, actualization of the collaborative governance model, and the sharing of experiences from the department's rich history and current practice that support patient advocacy.

The Personal Mastery Program

Personal Mastery—The Nurse as a Person, Colleague, and Integrator of Care is a three-day retreat in which nurses can come together to reflect on the art of nursing. They experience caring, healing of self and others, strengthening relationships, learning as a lifelong endeavor, and the joy and value of humor and lightheartedness in the work setting. Each nurse defines strategies to move his or her personal vision into practice.

On the first day of the retreat, participants focus on understanding themselves by identifying their personal visions and preferred work and learning styles; on exploring how to achieve a healthy balance of mind, body, and spirit; and on discussing how these factors influence their work with others. On the second day, the retreat centers on understanding others and the nursing profession, with participants exploring caring and curing behaviors from a nursing and a patient perspective. Patients also participate, sharing stories of what it was like to be patients and describing the systems and care they experienced. On the final day of the retreat, nurses concentrate on understanding the shared vision of the department, comparing their vision of professional practice to the shared vision of nursing practice at Abbott North-western. There is an emphasis on change mastery and developing a hardiness for change from a secure professional base.

In essence, personal mastery offers nurses protected time in a restful setting to reflect on the meaning of their practice through guided experiences. Participants are from all practice areas; and each group develops a charter for caring and has a six-month reunion.

Establishment of the Center for Professional and Clinical Development

In view of the changing health care environment and the need to focus on added value to patient care and practice, the role of the clinical education specialist at Abbott Northwestern was redefined. As a result, the Nursing Education Department became the Center for Professional and Clinical Development (the center), with a more clearly defined focus and an emphasis on reducing costs and improving clinical and professional practice.

The center provides education leadership and consultation for individuals, nursing units, and groups through three service areas:

1. *Professional development:* Several programs for professional development have been established. In addition to the Advocacy through Caring and Personal Mastery programs described earlier, these include Leadership Seminar—The Staff Nurse as Leader; Preceptor Development—Teacher and Coach; Coaching and Mentoring—A Guide for Nurse Leaders; Collaboration—Key to Quality and Innovation; and Development Opportunities—Organizational Leadership.
2. *Clinical development:* Orientation, competency-based practice, in-services, and mandatory education requirements.
3. *Learning services:* Conferences, recognition programs, outreach, writing and publishing, career guidance, academic alliances, individual consultation, and practice support.

The center is designed around learning, with emphasis on the professional accountability of each nurse to enhance patient care through active participation in the process of learning and its application to practice.

Emphasis on the application of learning at the point of care is based on this question: What are the clinical and professional skills and knowledge required to support patients/families through times of crisis or trauma associated with illness? Nurses' work also focuses on this question: What is required to maximize the patient's ability to return home with the optimal level of health and well-being?

As part of the department's philosophy, educators are understood to be enablers of learning rather than content experts. As such, they create an environment that provides a safe place for people to express diversity and increase understanding.

Practices of Exemplary Leaders

Kouzes's and Posner's work on practices of exemplary leaders is a useful framework for nurse leaders/consultants as they articulate their scope of practice and implement their role.[10] The practices of exemplary leaders are described as challenging the process, inspiring a shared vision, enabling others to act, modeling the way, and encouraging the heart. This has served to facilitate the developmental strategies for nurse leaders/consultants to increase their capacity to fulfill their roles.

A Comprehensive Curriculum for Quality Improvement

The consulting and development department created quality education/development building blocks to further the work of quality within nursing and to integrate nursing into the total quality environment. (See figure 4-5.) Programs and workshops were included to create competencies in self-knowledge, relationship versatility, cultural knowledge, process involvement, customer-focused work, team leadership, productive meetings, organizational alignment, systemic thinking, management skills, collaborative organizational design, and clinical process improvement.

Improved Labor–Management Relationships Based on a Professional Vision

Intentional relationship building occurred between the hospital and the Minnesota Nurses Association, the union representing staff nurses at Abbott Northwestern Hospital, to ensure the union had the respect and legitimacy it required to legally represent the nurses. Great care regarding inclusion, exploring common interests, and generating options to resolve issues, as well as a principle of "no surprises," guided the efforts. The search to identify common interests and engage in discussions of separate interests required practice and greater skill development. This effort resulted in greater creativity and flexibility with regard to options than had been possible previously, as well as greater understanding by management of union issues and greater appreciation by the union of management issues, interests, and requirements.

Implementation of the Clinical Practice Model

The clinical practice model is a system that supports the effective, individualized delivery of nursing care to patients based on their holistic care requirements and the art and science of professional nursing practice. (See figure 4-6.)

Figure 4-5. Quality Education/Development Building Blocks

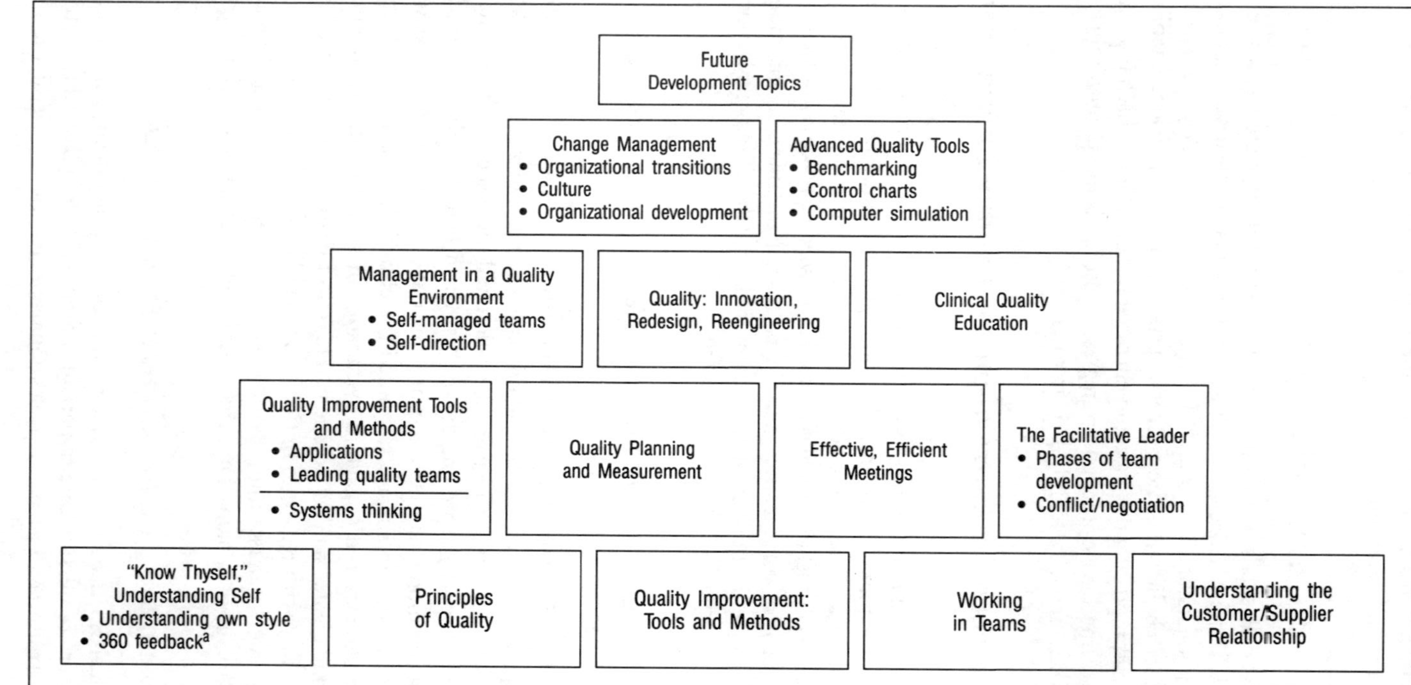

[a]*360 feedback* is a performance feedback method whereby an individual being evaluated receives feedback from his or her supervisor, peers, the people he or she supervises, and key customers.

Source: Used with permission of Abbott Northwestern Hospital, Minneapolis.

Figure 4-6.　Professional Practice Model

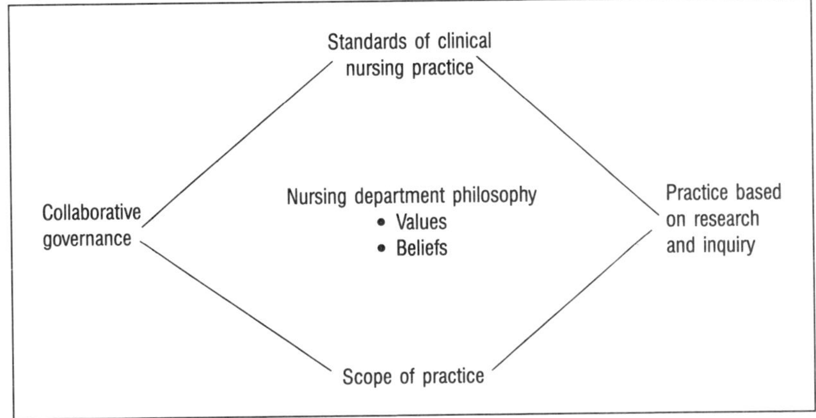

Source: Used with permission of Abbott Northwestern Hospital, Minneapolis.

Its goal is to define consistency in practice, ensure appropriateness of care, and decrease costs of care through increased efficiency, focus, and comprehensiveness. The model:

- Provides a framework for addressing the appropriateness, efficiency, and effectiveness of practice; aligns all of the activities in the department in a way that makes sense and strengthens nursing care delivery
- Reflects nursing department philosophy and standards
- Ties nursing to the work of the overall hospital and the managed care environment in which it exists
- Creates greater avenues for interdisciplinary, patient-focused collaboration

Implementation of a clinical practice model began when more than 80 nurses attended presentations on three professional practice models under consideration. The model that was selected originated from the Clinical Practice Model Resource Center in Grand Rapids, Michigan, with Bonnie Wesorick, founder and president. Implementation is expected to take 18 to 36 months. Of great value is that the model provides a common language and common performance standards and measurements—essential elements in creating a culture of high-quality practice.

Programs Designed to Respond to the Business Environment

Within the context of improved relations and skill enhancement, Abbott Northwestern launched a number of specific programs intended to respond to the new business environment. These included:

- A clinical nurse specialist group practice
- Nurse-to-nurse consultation
- The Hometown Nurse program
- Clinical nursing research

Clinical Nurse Specialist Group Practice

A multispecialty clinical nurse specialist (CNS) group practice was established to ensure coordination of patient care with maximum attention to quality and value. CNS group practice members partner with physician colleagues and collaborate with primary nurses, quality management specialists, and other members of the health care team to improve patient outcomes. They are population-based rather than unit- or program-based resources.

Previously, CNSs had been decentralized, reporting to divisional directors of nursing. There was a high variability in role implementation, and much of the role was focused toward support of projects, policies, and procedures. Now, CNSs provide nursing case management for high-risk patients, provide consultation and education on clinical issues of care, expand the use and development of clinical pathways for patient populations, and participate in interdisciplinary quality activities that address patient care issues.

Nurse-to-Nurse Consultation

Nurse-to-nurse consultation comprises a range of programs, products, and services designed to encourage nurses to share their expertise on clinical decision making and care delivery and to develop professional collaborative relationships to improve patient care. The program's goals are to create relationships and partnerships with nurses in rural communities, provide informational links for better continuity and patient-centered care, provide clinical and educational consultative services, and coordinate services at Abbott Northwestern for better access and use of resources. Program projects include an ongoing mechanism for monitoring calls to referring units, improvements in continuity of care on transfer and discharge, and creation of the *Nurse-to-Nurse Consultation Directory*, which includes an overview of 25 areas of nursing expertise, a listing of the nursing consultation services available in those areas, and the individuals available for consultation.

The Hometown Nurse Program

The Hometown Nurse program was created to promote sponsorship, a personalized environment, and continuity-of-care strategies for referral populations coming from regional settings to a hospital located in an urban environment. It helps out-of-state patients and their families feel more comfortable about being hospitalized far from home by linking them with nurses from the same hometown or region who can act as sponsors to help them navigate the intricacies of hospital care and the urban environment. In addition, the program links primary and tertiary care and builds relationships with patients, families, and health care professionals in both the hospital and the community. It recognizes the essential role of community care to patient outcomes. Program objectives are to create nurse partnerships among health care providers, to provide informational links for increased continuity and patient-centered care, and to create a hometown feel for patients hospitalized at Abbott Northwestern.

The Hometown Nurse program is an extension of Abbott Northwestern's care coordination, with 32 percent of the hospital's patient base being referred to Minneapolis from regional areas. It is now available to patients from 23 communities.

Clinical Nursing Research

The ultimate purpose of clinical nursing research at Abbott Northwestern Hospital is to promote scientific strategies to improve patient care. This represents a collaborative undertaking to bring nurse clinicians and scientists together at the patient bedside so that the practicing nurse can become a discriminate consumer of nursing research, use research findings in practice, and learn processes of clinical inquiry. This effort results in a data-based approach to nursing practice. A sense of inquiry, excitement, and intellectual challenge is present among the many nurses who participate directly or indirectly in these initiatives.

Nursing research ensures the attainment of new knowledge; creates a progressive, humanistic learning atmosphere; and values professional nursing practice. It helps nurses focus as one collaborative entity on the priority of nursing—patient care.

One successful nursing research project involved standardizing the approach to care for pressure ulcer patients, a vulnerable patient population. This standardization improved outcomes and reduced costs. The project resulted in savings of $50,000 over two months across seven patient care units. Ultimately, the project could save as much as $700,000 a year if implemented throughout the hospital.

Epicenters of Change

Throughout the past four years, within these overall departmental changes, patient care redesign has been occurring, supported in part by a grant from the Robert Wood Johnson Foundation/Pew Charitable Trusts called Strengthening Hospital Nursing: A Program to Improve Patient Care. In an environment of market-responsive change, it is a challenge to identify which change is the result of which stimulus. The grant work opened Abbott North-western's thinking to the larger community, reinforced partnerships with its customers, and was a catalyst to learning. The integration of quality, grant, strategic, and financial initiatives supported development of a more disciplined, results-oriented, customer-driven nursing department.

The grant sponsored three epicenters of change. These included:

1. Redesign of the rehabilitative care process
2. Redesign of the critical care process
3. Redesign of the cardiovascular care process

The methodology for work redesign was built on the foundation of collaborative governance, the Advocacy through Caring program, personal mastery, and the quality curriculum. The model used is an adaptation from the industrial reengineering work of Michael Hammer and the system-learning organization work of Peter Senge and Innovation Associates. (See figure 4-7.)

Nurses were among the process owners of these large system changes and worked with a design team to create the vision, design, and pilot for change. Targets were established, and results are being measured in the areas of:

- Improved clinical outcomes
- Increased patient/family satisfaction
- More meaningful work
- Increased efficiency of systems (for example, process simplification, reduced cycle times, and so on)
- Reduced costs

Figure 4-8 shows a model of the redesign team's organization.

Patients and payers were included on the design team as co-creators of change. The preliminary results are promising. Migrating from these epicenters are the extensions of innovation and CQI initiatives.

Innovations in infrastructure to support learning and change include personal mastery, team skills, curricula in CQI tools and methods, market/customer data feedback, and process owners and leaders.

Conclusion

Disciplines borrowed from business and industry, which were applied with full recognition of the mission, roles, and services of health care, have improved Abbott Northwestern's nursing department's focus and performance and have produced results. The key has been first "personalizing"

Figure 4-7. Innovation for Team Learning

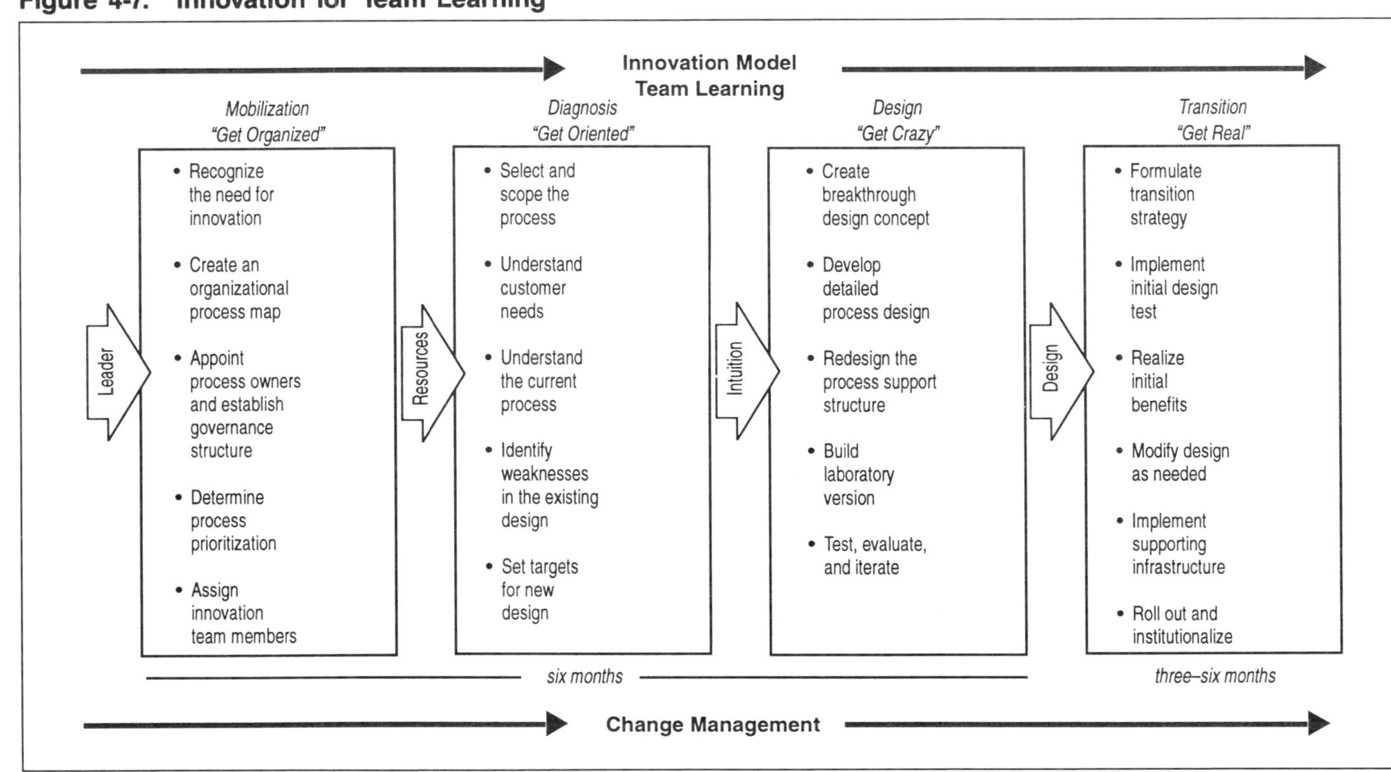

Figure 4-8.   Organizational Structure of the Nursing Department's Redesign Team

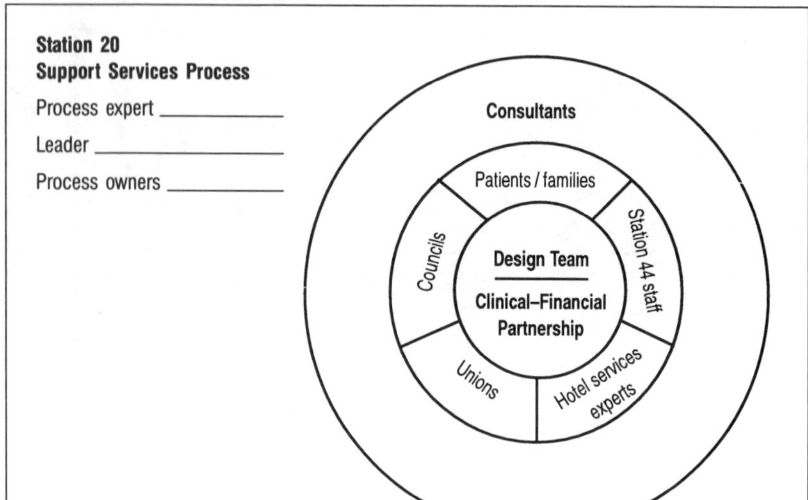

Source: Used with permission of Abbott Northwestern Hospital, Minneapolis.

the technologies and then applying them consistently. Identifying customer requirements, performance measures, and key organizational processes provided focus to the department's work. The capacity of the organization to improve and innovate was increased through development of internal consultants and experts who could lead personal mastery and change; teach and model the theory, tools, and methods of quality and reengineering; and create a culture of learning. Use of a patient-centered philosophy and vision grounded the nursing department in its purpose. Focus on the patient, involvement of stakeholders, and a grassroots approach to change have helped attenuate the fear often expressed in health care that use of business and industrial engineering practice in care delivery will result in a mechanistic, reductionistic, linear, by-the-numbers assembly-line environment for practice and will exclude the care provider's personal relationship with patients. However, the business discipline, when responding to customer/stakeholder requirements, can be liberating by providing focus and the technologies to realize that:

> Patients are the reason we exist.
> People are the reason we excel.
> Systems support the work.